Books by the Author:

Encyclopedia of Athletic Medicine (1972)
Dr. Sheehan on Running (1975)
Running and Being (1978)
Medical Advice for Runners (1978)

Dr. George Sheehan's

Medical Advice for Runners

By George A. Sheehan, M.D.

Dr. George Sheehan's

Medical Advice for Runners

By George A. Sheehan, M.D.

Recommended Reading:

Runner's World Magazine, $9.50/year
Box 366, Mountain View, CA 94042
Write for a free catalog of publications
and supplies for runners and other athletes.

World Publications, Mt. View, CA
Library of Congress 78-55788
ISBN 0-89037-134-2

Second Printing, November 1978

*"Strive to preserve your health,
and in this you will the better succeed
in proportion as you keep clear
of the physicians."*

Leonardo da Vinci

To all injured runners for their information, counsel and faith during this shared enterprise.

Contents

Introduction

"I do plead guilty to being fit, but only because at 44 I became bored with medicine. When I applied for the faculty at Rutgers Medical School, citing that boredom was my only qualification, the application was rejected. I then turned to a higher ambition to become a 44-year-old miler. And, in an absolute, unreasonable, single-minded dedication to that absurd project, discovered my body, my play, my vision and eventually a new life. I found my truth."

George A. Sheehan

The Rutgers medical faculty chose wisely. For in George Sheehan, they had met an unusual man—a man whose exceptional nature disqualified him from the study of the conventional, from diligent progress along the orthodox path of academic medicine. And for runners and their sport, it was a fortuitous decision. In the 16 years since he "pulled the emergency cord and ran out on the world," George Sheehan has discovered more than his own truth. He has become the sport's first doctor and its most eloquent philosopher, at once both proponent and defender of its faith. In the entire running fraternity, no one enjoys such respect, love and admiration.

It is not difficult to understand the appeal of George Sheehan.

He is loved for who he is, respected for all he has done for runners. At 5'10" and 135 pounds, he is the archtypical long-distance runner. Quiet, undemonstrative, emotionally reserved, he is visibly fragile—"too brittle for direct fighting, too exposed to thrive in the over-stimulation of ordinary social life." So it is in the solitude of the road, away from the contemporary bustle, that he communicates with himself; here that he has discovered himself and his truth.

Through his rare ability to describe the essence of that conversation, we learn who he is and what running means to him. We catch a glimpse of the warmth, the uninhibited wisdom, the total self-acceptance that make him so unusual.

"Running made me free," he writes. "It rid me of concern for the opinion of others, dispensed me from rules and regulations imposed from outside. Running let me start from scratch. Running was discovery, a return to the past, a proof that life did come full circle and the child was father to the man. Because the person I found, the self I discovered, was the person I was in my youth—the person who was hypersensitive to pain, both physical and psychic, a nominal coward; the person who did not wish his neighbor ill but did not wish him well either. That person was me and always had been."

In becoming himself, in recovering the freedom and individuality of his youthful self, George Sheehan unlocked the treasure that we now share—a tireless, inconquerable spirit and a restless, insatiable mind.

"My instinct is to fight, to persevere, to push against resistance and to take the path least traveled," he says.

It is to this personal ethic that runners are the most indebted, for it is the source of this book and the inspiration that has established the core and the ethos of running medicine. For George Sheehan was the first doctor to rank his own profession, medicine, alongside the dog and the motor car as the three natural enemies of the runner. And having admitted that, he did something about it.

Personal experience of injury—"I became a mobile medical museum, a clinical exhibit of the illnesses of the long-distance runner"—taught him that those charged with the care of athletes were unable to cope with his running problems. The only solution would be to find the answers himself. In defiance of rigid scientific principles, he began his "experiment of one" on the road, his laboratory. Personal observation led him to conclude that the special feature of running injuries was that they resulted from factors intrinsic to the body. ("Eventually, I took a biblical approach to these afflictions. The cause of man's infirmity is to be found in man himself.") Each athlete, he concluded, was born with built-in weaknesses which training and the environment would ruthlessly expose. Finally, he proposed a revolutionary concept: that the crux of the injury problem begins at the interface between the foot and the running surface.

With typical self-deprecation, he still denies any knowledge of how the running foot functions. But the experts in this field acknowledge George as the inspiration behind and the relentless champion of sports podiatry.

His contributions do not end with philosophy and feet—the two extremes, you might say, of the runner's well-being. This book and all his writings provide a synthesis of the totality of running medicine, his subject, the subject which he has pioneered, fathered, enriched and which will always bear the stamp of his individual creativity, insight and understanding.

Quite fittingly, it may be Emerson's description of the ideal man that most nearly captures the attributes, the contributions, the person of George Sheehan:

"A brave and upright man who must find or cut a straight road to everything excellent in the earth, and not only go honorably himself but make it easier for all who follow him to go in honor and with benefit."

Tim Noakes, M.D.
Cape Town, South Africa.

Foreword

After I read Tom Osler's *Serious Runner's Handbook*, I called him. "This is going to be a classic," I said, "except for one chapter. The one on injuries is terrible."

There was silence on the other end. Tom is a thinker and not given to a quick reply.

I finally asked him, "Have you ever been injured?"

"Hardly ever," he replied.

This book, then, is the companion piece to Tom Osler's. His contains the best practical advice on training and racing you will find anywhere, because Tom is a master at that. Here, you will find what I am master at—injuries.

I am made out of what, in medical school, we called P.P.P. (piss-poor protoplasm). There is hardly an injury I have not experienced, hardly a weakness known to the body that is not resident in mine—or if not in mine, then not farther than my kitchen table where I receive the complaints of my dozen children, nine of whom are runners and two are basketball players.

We Sheehans not only hand down clothing, we hand down crutches, casts, foot supports, knee braces and other surgical supplies. The most asked-for item in the house after the butter is the adhesive tape. My one non-running daughter is thinking of joining another clan.

But if you would be an authority on any injury or illness, the best way is to have it yourself. That is the only way to be an expert.

My father, who was a heart specialist, once had a heart attack victim stop him in mid-question and say, "But how would you know? You've never had a heart attack."

It is not entirely necessary, I'm sure, but I know you become much more perceptive after you have been a patient. After my bout with hepatitis, I was able to diagnose it over the phone, usually by the end of the second sentence. Telephone diagnosis is a rare aptitude usually found only in maiden aunts with certain clairvoyant powers.

The same thing happened with gall bladder disease. After I discovered I had gallstones (and not a recurrent ulcer as I suspected) and had surgery, I became a whiz at picking up the gall bladder vibes.

And so it goes down the line if you've had it. If you've been there and back, you have an advantage no end of book-learning can erase.

I did not suspect when I came back to running at the age of 45 that I would be able to make any contribution to the sport. Now, I know I was wrong. What new runners wanted most was not records or even personal bests. They did not want anything but to keep running.

So what runners needed was somebody to do patrol duty—to get all the disorders and learn how to deal with them. The days of 10- and 20- and 30-mile-a-day training were at hand, bringing with them overuse problems in every system of the body. Someone had to suffer so later generations of runners could run easier.

When I began, we runners were a handful. I have a picture of my first New York Marathon. The entire field is no larger than a football squad. I remember that day well, because I broke a shoestring right on the starting line. Everyone waited while I got another one and put it in my shoe. That day, I knew my career would be in incurring misfortune and learning how to deal with it.

I made steady progress, from then on going from one injury to another, learning what to do and what not to do, learning who could help and who couldn't, learning how to survive that dreadful period when running was impossible.

There came a time when I learned too much. For almost three years, I went without injury. Then, I became the victim of shoe manufacturers' largess: free shoes. I left my trusty Tigers, bought originally because they were half the price of anything else. Soon, I was into a variety of problems spawned by these new, presumably better shoes. A new world had opened up.

With my tissues, the prospects are limitless. "There is a crack in everything God made," said Emerson. Mine are wide and numerous. I have no worry that things will get better, that my career of illness and injury is drawing to a close. I have only to redouble my efforts, and some new, interesting and altogether engrossing overuse problem will come along.

There are some things I have yet to experience—the thrill of passing blood after a long race, the effort migraine, groin pain. But perhaps they are in my future.

Some of my running friends say they will donate their bodies to science after they die. I have done it while I'm still alive. What I have done best is get injured and suffer. I have learned to be a running doctor by being a runner first and a doctor second. Therefore, much of what I say here goes beyond or defies the conventional medical wisdom I once accepted.

George A. Sheehan, M.D.
Red Bank, N.J.
July 1978

From the Publisher
who brings you
Dr. Sheehan each month

PART ONE:
SPORTS MEDICINE

"Treat the reason, not the result.
Treat the cause, not the effect."

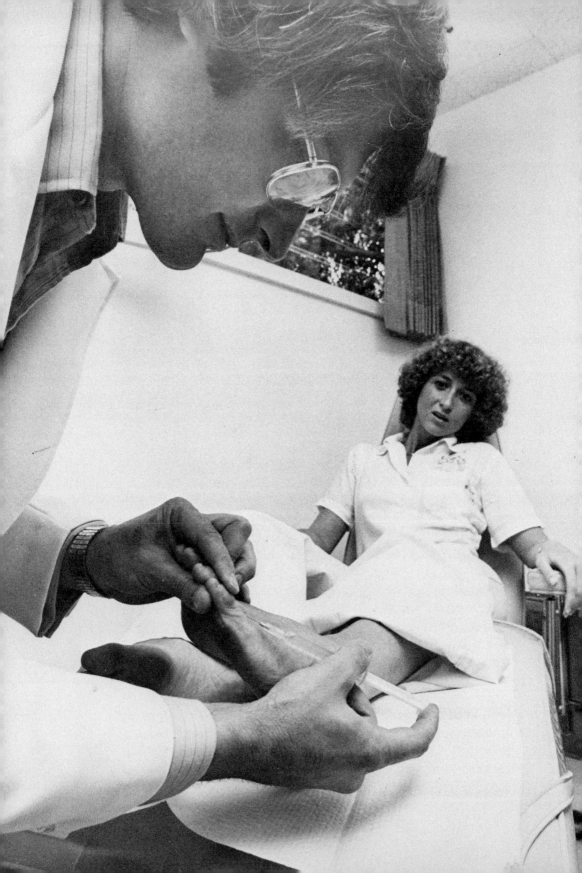

Chapter 1
Diseases of Excellence

When we hear the word "athlete," we immediately think of someone who is performing at his maximum, someone who has reached excellence in his chosen sport. And that is indeed the definition proposed by Professor C. T. Mervyn Davies of the London School of Hygiene and Tropical Medicine. "An athlete," says Professor Davies, "is someone who makes maximum use of his genetic endowment through training in his environment."

The athlete's formula for excellence, therefore, is *genes plus training plus environment.* And this formula, being the source of his excellence, is also the source of his "diseases of excellence," the varieties of overuse syndromes I deal with in this book.

The major part of athletic ability is inherent. It has been said that if you wish to be an Olympic champion or a world record-holder, you must choose your parents well. Dr. Roger Bannister, the first sub-four-minute miler, said that about one person in a hundred is a "motor genius," and added that the limiting factor in performance is the amount of training a person will accept. The implication was that the limit would have to be something acceptable to a person's psyche and to his conception of how he should best live his life. However, it is apparent now that the limitation is the point of breakdown of the organism. Athletes, whether they are motor geniuses or not, simply multiply their training until disability occurs.

11

Studies show an astounding increase in training quantity and quality since World War II. Nowadays, teenage runners are training at distances unheard of for champion runners in 1930. Running 50 miles a week is now considered quite ordinary, and some marathoners regularly run 50-200 miles a week. Training includes high-speed anaerobic work as well, and this seems to have a special type of stress quite beyond the time and distance put into it.

Finally, the environment, which includes shoes, surfaces, meteorological conditions, diet, sleep and other day-to-day activities, has contributed more and more to the stresses applied to the athlete. Therefore, we must take into account the entire milieu of the athlete, as well as his training program and constitutional attributes, in diagnosing and treating his illnesses.

All of this is easily recognizable as the "holistic" approach to the patient that was urged upon us in medical school. We have gotten away from that approach, but nothing less will work in treating the athlete. When he comes into your office, you must begin at the beginning, and try to know him and how he trains. You must not neglect looking at his shoes, finding what he wears in a race versus what he wears in practice, which side of the road he runs on, and whether he trains on hills or level ground. These are all vital to the diagnosis and, therefore, to the treatment. Unless you consider all three aspects—genes, training and environment—you will probably fail in the treatment of this patient.

But let us go back to the beginning: These diseases of excellence always (if one can ever say "always") begin with an inherent constitutional defect. When you run 100 miles a week, you find it. Whatever system breaks down, wherever the athlete begins to give way, there will be behind it some inherent weakness. This can be seen in any body system, but the musculoskeletal system can be seen as the prototype.

Analyze any runner with an overuse injury of the lower extremity, and you will discover he has a structural problem, usually one of the following:

1. *Biomechanically weak feet.* This is usually a "Morton's foot" with the short big toe and the long second toe. This foot pronates (rolls inward) abnormally due to laxity along the first

metatarsal segment. Any other pronatory influence can do the same thing, however. The excessively high-arched "cavus" foot is also at hazard.

2. *Leg-length discrepancy.* Shortening, usually of the non-dominant leg, causes a variety of symptoms, mainly in the low back and upper leg.

3. *Minor abnormalities of the lower back area.*

The runner with one or more of these constitutional problems superimposes the effects of training. When you train, three things happen to your muscles; two are bad. Training improves muscle efficiency for the activity in question. But at the same time, the prime-movers are overdeveloped, and get tighter and less flexible; the antagonists become relatively weak. Eventually, a muscle pulls. In a weak muscle, this occurs in its belly. A strong muscle that pulls usually does so at its musculo-tendinous junction or at its bony attachment.

But overdeveloped prime-movers and weak antagonists do more than pull muscles. They cause further pronation at foot-strike, and thereby increase the tendency toward problems in the foot, leg and knee. At the same time, they increase mis-alignment at the lumbar area, creating low-back and sciatic difficulties.

Finally, the environment comes into play. Some shoes fail to handle impact or the pronatory influences. Slanted surfaces caused increased pronation. Running against traffic, for instance, will increase pronation in the right foot and cause symptoms. Therapeutic orthotics (custom-made shoe inserts) themselves may cause difficulty because they overcorrect the inherent constitutional weakness.

At *Runner's World,* we conducted a poll and more than 1000 runners responded to questions on injuries involving their running. Of the total, 60% said that they had been injured for a considerable length of time. Those injuries and their incidence are shown in Table One. When we analyzed these by age, sex, mileage and racing or non-racing participation, we received the information in Table Two.

Unfortunately, overuse syndromes in other systems have not been studied quite so closely and have not been so well documented. However, I know from answering runners' questions over a period of eight years that the other systems share in this phenomenon.

TABLE ONE					
Knee	23.2%	Hip	7.9%	Ankle	6.7%
Shin	14.6%	Thigh	7.5%	Arch	4.2%
Achilles	12.4%	Calf	7.0%	Groin	2.2%
Forefoot	8.3%	Heel	7.0%		

Results of a poll of over 1000 respondents, of whom 60% reported prolonged injuries

TABLE TWO			
VARIABLE	**INJURY RATE**	**VARIABLE**	**INJURY RATE**
Age		**Years Running**	
< 19 years old	72%	< 5	63%
> 40 years old	57%	5-9	52%
		> 9	56%
Sex			
Female	90%	**Racing**	
Male	60%	Yes	65%
		No	27%
Mileage			
> 50 miles/wk.	73%	**Surface**	
< 25 miles/wk.	34%	No difference between hard surface and soft, but more minor problems with hard.
Result of a poll of over 1000 respondents.			

In the gastro-intestinal system, the runners' main complaints seem to be cramps and diarrhea. It is my impression that training brings to light underlying, previously asymptomatic tendencies and weaknesses much the same as it does in the musculo-skeletal system. So here we must consider lactase deficiency, gluten sensitivity, irritable colon, weak esophageal sphincter, diverticulitis and ulcer susceptibility. Any of these diseases can be taken from a latent state to active illness by overracing or overtraining.

We can see similar problems in every other system. The heart is certainly affected. Rhythm disturbances and abnormal EKGs abound. The heart also enlarges. Resultant EKGs can sometimes bewilder the physician and wrongly cause him to terminate an athlete's career.

The respiratory system is not exempt. Exercise-induced asthma is a continuing mystery, but probably is due in part to faulty breathing mechanics and air-trapping.

And so it goes. I have seen people run themselves into an agitated depression, develop blood in the urine, and be treated for pseudo-anemia that appeared as training progressed.

Finally, we are faced with the problems of staleness or exhaustion, the final indignity to the distance runner. Having found this sport and escaped injury, he finds his pursuit of excellence stymied by exhaustion. And he discovers that no one knows exactly what it is or what is at its root. As yet, we have no way of knowing when a runner is exactly at peak and, therefore, only a razor's edge from disaster.

The distance runner achieves excellence by making the most of his genetic endowment through training in his environment. This formula for greatness is also the cause of his diseases of excellence. The physician must take a holistic view of this illness and act accordingly.

Chapter 2
What Doctors Can Do

NEW SPORTS MEDICINE

The new sports medicine is a development of the new athlete. The athlete of the 1970s is the common man and woman engaging in what were previously called "minor" sports: sports like running that involve innumerable repetitions of the same action.

Athletes in these sports require medical care profoundly different from the collision sports that previously occupied the doctor's time. In those major sports, the care is simply the treatment of trauma transplanted from the emergency room to the playing field.

The new sports medicine is orthopedic *medicine,* not orthopedic *surgery.* It is concerned with balance and architecture, with structural integrity and postural stability. The major advances, therefore, have not been in drugs or surgical procedures. They have been in biomechanics—that is, in the re-establishment of body physics and the avoidance of surgery.

A few years back, sports medicine was still a surgical speciality. The typical patient was one of Saturday's heros, and the typical injury was the damage resulting from a split-second collision of the irresistible force and the immovable object. The treatment, almost inevitably, was surgery.

"The sports medicine meetings I attended," a team physician told me at that time, "are really surgical conferences." He had been trained, he said, in the traditional approach: Make the diagnosis and select the suitable operation.

But even then, the handwriting was on the wall. There were no longer appropriate operations. We had gone from the sports medicine of trauma to the sports medicine of overuse. We had come to the "diseases of excellence"—those incurred simply by doing too much for too long a time.

The typical patient had become a common, garden-variety human being engaged in a non-contact sport. The typical injury resulted from innumerable repetitions of the same action. The typical treatment became medical.

The problem, you see, became too much conditioning, not too little; over-developed muscles rather than under-developed ones. The basic cause was a structural weakness in the body, compounded by the effects of training and equipment, rather than a momentary cataclysmic reaction between two opposing forces.

The major advances in sports medicine have, therefore, been in the field of biomechanics. Two particular innovations stand out.

First is the idea of strength/flexibility balance. We had always thought strength to be necessary, but it is only in the past few years that flexibility has received the attention it deserves. Flexibility not only is necessary to prevent muscle pulls, strains and tears, but it also prevents abnormal stress in the arch of the foot, shoulder, elbow and other structures involved in sports movement.

The second major advance was the birth of sports podiatry. Podiatrists who specialized in the diagnosis and treatment of foot disorders finally came into their own when runners discovered that the foot could cause troubles in the leg, knee, thigh and even low back. Study of the biomechanics of the running foot has led to competent care of previously intractable disorders of the foot and lower extremity.

Unfortunately, in the minds of many doctors orthodoxy still prevails. The new athlete and the new sports medicine have not been matched by the new sports physician. When that happens, athletes frequently resort to "fringe medicine"—that is, they go looking for cures elsewhere.

They should be warned that this can also be a dead end. To be sure, many of these things work. Acupuncture, for instance, is effective in that it relieves discomfort. However, it doesn't correct the basic difficulties in the architecture.

What ever is done for an overuse syndrome must deal with the reason, not the result; the cause—not the effect. And that is what the new sports medicine—strength/flexibility balance and sports podiatry—does so well.

SPECIALISTS

Q: I have a number of foot and leg injuries, and have had conflicting advice from an orthopedic surgeon, a podiatrist and a chiropractor. The surgeon suggested I change my sport. The podiatrist gave me shoe inserts, which the chiropractor said were making my problems worse. What should I do?

A: Conflicting advice is all the athlete ever gets. Every health care professional—physician, podiatrist, chiropractor—is a little king. Each sits in his office and pontificates. I know, because I do it myself.

What the athlete needs is a primary care physician who is himself an athlete. He would be able to act as the athlete's representative and select among, or integrate, the proposed therapies. In other words, he would stand between the athlete and these specialists and their competing disciplines.

That is the problem. They should be cooperating instead of competing. Until this utopia arrives, my advice is to stay with the podiatrist. Whatever has to be done will have to start with your feet. He may not have done it correctly yet, but give him another chance.

ORTHOPEDISTS VS. PODIATRISTS

Q: I am an orthopedic surgeon, and as such I have been embarrassed at one time or another in virtually all of your columns, as well as your books. Why have you categorically branded us as totally ineffective in the care of runners and dogmatically advised your readers to shun orthopedists in favor of podiatrists?

Your criticisms of orthopedists may have been valid a few years ago, but they are not any longer. Within our profession,

there has been a great upsurge of interest in the study of biomechanics and clinical problems of the runner. Most of us in
sports medicine, by virtue of the increasing volume of patients
with running-related problems in our offices, are honestly trying
to come to grips with the basic anatomical variations predis-
posing to injury; we are not simply injecting cortisone and
advising people to quit running.

You universally advise your readers to seek a podiatrist to
cure their ailing knees and feet. Yet a good sports podiatrist
knowledgeable in runners' problems is as rare as a knowledgeable orthopedist.

Podiatrists, by virtue of their specialty, are limited in their
knowledge of the human body, and most of them do not even
pretend to understand all the forces about the back, hips and
knees, much less the effect of the foot on these forces. Moreover,
their prices are outlandish. They routinely charge $150-200 for the
same arch supports I get for my patients for $25.

A: I think you are right in suggesting that many podiatrists
do a bad job of handling runners. I emphasize that in talking to
podiatrists.

A good sports podiatrist is a pearl in a running community.
If he is a runner himself, so much the better. A bad podiatrist is
more than a failure for the runners he is treating. In addition,
he damns podiatry, a key specialty in the treatment of overuse
problems.

Podiatrists are, of course, only part of the total cure. Athletes
should have a team of specialists, but there is no team. What
actually happens is that the first specialist seen captures the
athlete. There is no communication or consultation coopera-
tion. Until such teamwork occurs, the one specialist most likely
to succeed is the sports podiatrist.

THE MANIPULATORS

Q: What is your opinion of osteopaths and chiropractors?
Also, what do you think of acupuncture and acupressure?

A: Osteopaths and chiropractors have much to offer. They
can manipulate, for instance—a mode of therapy usually
ignored by orthopedic surgeons. They are also quite good at

discovering limb-length discrepancy, a major factor in many resistant back injuries.

Furthermore, chiropractors do not dispense drugs, a fact which puts them on their mettle to produce results in a natural way. However, they tend to go overboard on nutrition because of this.

I think that acupuncture and acupressure work, but only temporarily. They do not correct the cause of the problem. Like drugs, they treat the effect.

ACUPRESSURE

Q: Why do you bother to comment on hogwash such as acupressure? At best, it does little harm, since well-informed people just dismiss it as the product of a colossal ignorance. At worst, it prevents recourse to competent medical help, and that can be serious.

A: The fact that it is difficult to explain how a therapy works or that indeed the practitioners of such therapies invent a whole new language is not enough to discredit it.

This is not to say that I think them important to athletes. They offer symptomatic relief only and, therefore, differ only in degree from butazolidine and cortisone shots.

My 15 years in running have taught me to go to the cause of the problem. Other therapies simply delay getting back to pain-free running.

"The truth is what works," said James. Runners usually have to find that out for themselves. Advocacy of this kind at least makes a dent in medical orthodoxy and causes the athlete to consider alternative modes of therapy.

PART TWO: RUNNING FITNESS

"All we need to know is the fitness equation:
How fast? How far? How often?"

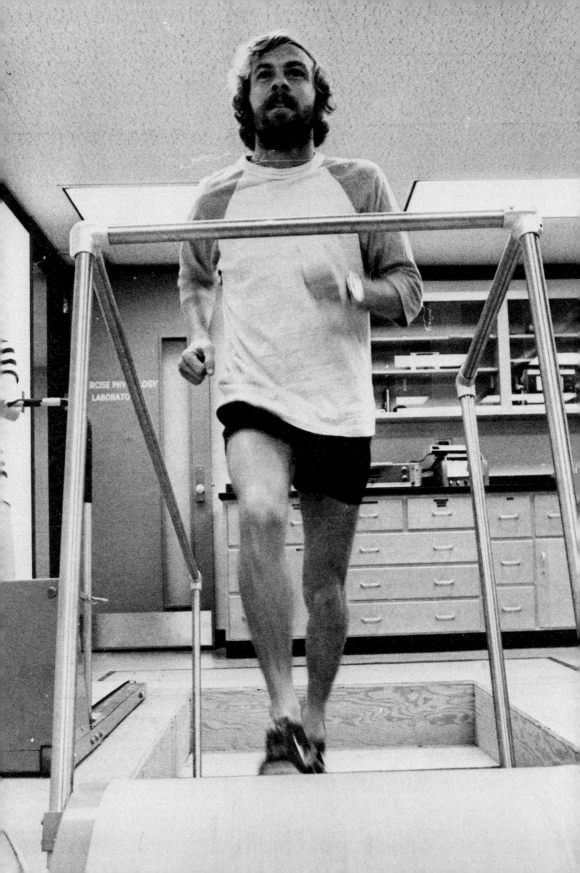

Chapter 3
Reasons to Run

I am 15 years a distance runner and still trying to explain this self-renewing inner compulsion. The more I run, the more I want to run. The more I run, the more I live a life conditioned and influenced and fashioned by my running. And the more I run, the more certain I am that I am heading for my real goal: to become the person I am.

In the beginning, I never suspected this would happen. I began running for the usual reasons: to get in shape but really to improve my appearance rather than my wind, and then to prevent a heart attack and add some years to my life. I learned by rote the good things running would do for my cholesterol and my coronary arteries, how my blood pressure would go down and my energy would increase.

I began as all of us should. First, I did "scout pace"—50 steps jogging alternating with 50 steps walking; five minutes at first and then each day a little more, all done at a speed which would allow me to talk with a companion. Later, it became all running, and I reached 30 minutes a day. Finally, I reached an hour every other day. I had become a runner.

By then, all my original reasons had disappeared in my wake. I had no further use for them. They reminded me of what Ronald Knox had written about proofs of the existence of God. They were only scaffolding, he said, and when your faith had been constructed, they were no longer necessary. They could be discarded and forgotten.

Running, I saw, was more than fitness and longevity. It was more than health and a trim body. Running was more than weight lost and muscles revived. Running was a total experience. It became part of my lifestyle.

If Bacon had written on running, he would have put it this way: "Running maketh the whole man." I see that whole person as being part animal, part child, part artist and part saint. Running makes me all of these. It makes me a whole person.

I began as body. "Be first a good animal," wrote Emerson. I am. I have that animal energy, that ease of movement, that good tight body, that sense of occupying just the right amount of space. I am pared down to bone and muscle. My skin taut, my eyes clear, I have become my body. I occupy it with delight.

The tests prove what I feel. My biological age is that of a person 30 years younger. I have the oxygen capacity and physical work capacity of a 28-year-old instead of someone approaching 60. My pulse is slow, my blood pressure normal, my body fat a mere 5%. Yet I am no different from others my age who run with me. Running proves that man at any age is the greatest marvel in the world.

Next comes the child. Running makes me a child, a child at play. That is the aim of life: to become an adult while still remaining a child at heart. Play is the key. There, we do things because we want to, without thought of payment.

Play is something we would do for nothing, something that has meaning but no purpose. When I run, I feel that. For that hour a day, I am a child finally doing what I want to do and enjoying it. When I do, I realize what happens to the body is simply a bonus. I must first play an hour a day, then all other things will be added.

One great addition is to make myself an artist. Being an artist is, after all, only seeing things as if for the first time. When we do, we see the real meaning of things, the solutions to our problems. Running gives me that creativity. It provides the meditative setting. It opens up areas in my mind I seem not to use otherwise.

At a minimum, it places me where these things can happen. A physician friend of mine expressed it this way: "I decided to run at a pace that would allow me to (1) enjoy my surroundings; (2) let me think a bit; (3) be alone for an hour a day." I agree.

On the roads, at a pace I could run forever, I find what that "forever" is all about.

Finally, running has given me a chance to be a saint, to be a hero. Like everyone else, I want to be challenged. I want to find out whether or not I am a coward. I want to see how much effort I can put out...what I can endure...if I measure up. Running allows that.

I can run the classic race, the mile, and know the terrible pain that accompanies the third quarter-mile and the almost total oblivion of the final hundred yards to the finish. I can suffer, die and be born again in a six-mile race over hills on a cross-country course. And I can compete with myself in the marathon, the race Roger Bannister called the "acme of athletic heroism."

There are as many reasons for running as there are days in the year, years in my life. But mostly I run because I am an animal and a child, an artist and a saint. So, too, are you. Find your own play, your own self-renewing compulsion, and you will become the person you are meant to be.

Chapter 4
How to Start Running

SEVEN RULES

The "golden rules" of good health and long life have not changed since Hippocrates. Our days and their enjoyment are measured by following seven commonsense commandments:

1. *Don't smoke.*
2. *Get seven hours of sleep.*
3. *Eat breakfast.*
4. *Keep your weight down.*
5. *Drink alcoholic beverages moderately.*
6. *Exercise regularly.*
7. *Don't eat between meals.*

Dean Breslow and associates at the UCLA School of Public Health have studied what happened to people who kept or broke these rules. Their investigation came up with some interesting findings. A person who followed six of the seven rules had an 11 years longer life expectancy at age 45 than those who followed less than four rules. And a 75-year-old who followed the prescription to the letter had the same physical health status as those aged 35-44 who followed less than three.

As you can see, exercise is important to vitality and longevity, but it doesn't stand alone.

DEFINING FITNESS

Q: What is physical fitness, and how do we attain it? Why is running a good way to become fit?

A: Physical fitness is the capacity to carry out everyday activities without excessive fatigue and with enough reserve energy to enjoy your leisure time.

It is generally agreed that aerobic endurance activity, exercise done on a pay-as-you-go basis as far as oxygen is concerned, is the best way to become fit. One of the best aerobic activities is running.

Running is open to almost everyone. It requires a minimum of equipment and no special facilities. It can be done alone, anywhere, anytime. A maximum return is available in a minimum amount of time.

After 6-8 weeks of training, you can expect to see, among other things: a slower heart rate, increased heart stroke volume, lowered blood pressure, lowering of the cholesterol, increase in high-density lipoproteins (now thought to provide protection against coronary disease), weight loss, increased work capacity, increased lean body weight.

And there are psychological benefits: Running provides contemplation, conversation, and competition—all of which give an added dimension to our lives. Running also improves the self-image, makes for better coping ability, lowers anxiety and is helpful in fighting depression.

BEGINNING

Q: Would you briefly list guidelines a beginner should follow in order to start running safely and to keep going?

A: Before starting, assess your physical condition. If you are over 40, or have a family history of heart disease, a "stress test" is recommended. This treadmill test spots heart irregularities during exercise monitored by an electrocardiograph. If necessary, exercise limits are set by the physician.

The goal of a running program is first to improve your cardio-vascular endurance. That is, through training, you maximize the transport of oxygen throughout the body. Your primary concern when training is not speed but time spent running. This "aerobic" or endurance activity trains the heart and lungs as well as the muscles.

Your schedule should call for at least four runs each week. Each should be 10-15 minutes to start; anything less has little aerobic effect. During these runs (or a mixture of walking and running, if necessary), your pulse should rise to 60-80% of maximum. That's usually 135-150 beats per minute.

Whatever your level of fitness, your training motto should be: "Train, don't strain." Take the "talk test" while running. If you're breathing too hard to carry on a conversation, you're going too fast.

It is also wise to adopt the "hard-easy" principle of training when planning your workouts. That is, alternate a hard workout with an easy one. For your initial workouts, you may want to alternate a day of running with a day of walking, or you may need a day of rest between workouts. To maintain regular running, you must avoid injury and staleness.

Start by dressing properly. In warm weather, loose-fitting shirts and shorts work best. The goal is to keep the body cool. Liquids should be taken *before and during* your runs. Eight to ten ounces every 20 minutes is sufficient.

During cold weather, dress in layers. This traps heat. Start with wool next to the body; it is a good insulator, even when wet. Use it to cover the head (where 40% of body heat escapes), hands and feet. Long-johns are good for the legs. Wear a couple of shirts, and cover them with a nylon parka to further trap heat. One or more layers may be removed as you warm up.

The most important part of a runner's gear is the running shoes. Check for good cushioning (for shock absorption), flexibility at the front (to prevent shin splints), built-up heel (to protect the Achilles tendons) and a strong heel counter (to keep the feet stable on impact). The shoes should feel good right away, without having to be "broken in."

The importance of foot and leg care cannot be underestimated. Statistics show that two of every three runners suffer an injury in this area.

One major cause of injuries is muscle imbalance. The muscles in the back of the body which help the legs move become tight from running. Conversely, the muscles in the front become weak from inactivity. To solve this imbalance, the tight muscles must be stretched, the weak muscles must be strengthened. Ten minutes of exercises before or after you run (or both) is advised.

To complete your warmup, after doing the exercises, jog slowly until you break into a sweat. This usually happens after 6-10 minutes. By starting slowly, you reduce the risk of injuries.

Another cause of injury is improper footstrike. When running a mile, the runner's foot strikes the ground about 1000 times. So check your form. You should run erect, with the foot landing under the torso. The foot should land almost flat, slightly back toward the heel. And the knee should be slightly bent on contact.

Check your running surface. If you run on the roads (face traffic for safety), the grade or slope may strain your leg. Roads may be too hard on some people. They should try running on grass or dirt. On the other hand, these surfaces may be too uneven for certain runners. They should switch to smooth roads.

Check your shoes regularly. Wornout shoes must be rebuilt or replaced before they cause injuries.

Lastly, check the feet. They may be weak or imbalanced because of a second toe longer than the big toe (Morton's foot syndrome). They may be at the end of one leg which is shorter than the other. The help of a sports podiatrist (foot specialist) can be invaluable.

A PROGRAM

Q: Please give specifics for setting up a running program—how much to run, how fast and how often?

A: Our fancy often turns to dreams of past glories, to those years when our bodies did our will. The morning air, the bright sun, the green trees recall days when only darkness could end our play. We were giants—if not in strength at least in endurance. We knew what it was like to be a good animal. And we wonder if we could ever be that way again.

The answer, of course, is yes. We can walk or job or run our way back to those days, those joys, that level of fitness. All we need to know is the fitness equation, the answers to the questions: How fast? How far? How often?

HOW FAST?

Few people know how fast to train. Most assume they must punish themselves to become fit. They think that becoming an athlete is hard work. It just isn't so. Fitness must be fun. The rule again is: "Train, don't strain." So the pace for fitness should be comfortable and enjoyable. Effort should be the measure, not speed, and your body should tell you your proper pace, not the stopwatch.

I use the word "pace" deliberately. It is a better word than "speed." Speed has to do with numbers, statistics, minutes per mile. Pace has to do with feelings and is not a matter of precise mathematics. It has to do with adjectives like "easy" and "breathless" and "headlong." But the adjective we are looking for is "comfortable," and we find it by asking our bodies.

This seemingly unscientific idea has a solid scientific basis in the theory of perceived exertion. Proposed by Gunnar Borg in 1960, it states that the effort perceived by the body is almost identical to that recorded by a machine. Borg discovered that body perception is, in fact, superior to any single physiological determination.

PERCEIVED EXERTION AND PULSE RATE		
Borg Scale		**Pulse**
6-7	(very, very light)	60-70
8-9	(very light)	80-90
10-11	(fairly light)	100-110
12	(comfortable pace)	120
13-14	(somewhat hard)	130-140
15-16	(hard)	150-160
17-18	(very hard)	170-180
19-20	(very, very hard)	190-200

The Borg Scale starts at six (very, very light) and ends up at 20 (very, very hard). Adding a zero to the rating gives the usual pulse rate at that level of activity. The walker, jogger or runner, therefore, aims at the mid-range between light and hard, the area we perceive to be comfortable. This is a pace at which we could hold a conversation with a companion—the "talk test."

Now, you might say that you couldn't run across the room without becoming short of breath. Then don't. Begin by walking and then work up to the scout-pace (alternating 50 steps walking and 50 steps running). Finally, you will be able to run continually, in comfort. You will be able to put yourself on "automatic pilot" and enjoy your thoughts and the countryside.

Listen to your body. Do not be a blind and deaf tenant. Hear what your muscles and heart and lungs are telling you. Above all, get in union with your body. Ride yourself as a jockey does a horse, finally becoming one with it.

There will come times when the sheer joy of this mysterious fusion, this wholeness will drive you to see just what you can do. But this is unnecessary, for you now have the pace. Do not push. You have found the groove. Stay in it.

Even when you have become proficient, and the comfortable pace becomes faster and faster, you still must do the first 6-10 minutes very slowly. You must allow the juices to flow, the temperature to rise, the circulation to adapt. You must give the body time to make all those marvelous, intricate adjustments that happen when you finally set yourself in motion. When you do, you will experience that warm sweat that comes with the onset of second-wind and get the feeling that you just might spend the rest of the day running.

When I get into that second-wind, I settle down to my comfortable pace and let the body do the thinking. My ground speed varies with the time of day (early-morning runs take one minute a mile longer) or with heat and humidity, but effort does not vary. The identical thing happens when I run against a headwind or up hills, or on those days when I am upset psychologically. But whether the watch says 8 minutes a mile or 10, the pace is the same. It is comfortable, and because my perceived exertion is always the same, the effort is identical and the physiological benefits are identical as well.

Once you have begun this way, success is assured. There is no need to rush, no need to hurry. Nor is there any need to worry. When you run at a comfortable pace, you are well within your physical limits. ("I have never been harmed," said Montaigne, "by anything that was a real pleasure.")

Find the comfortable pace and enjoy it. Fitness is bound to follow.

HOW FAR?

Again, we must consult the body. The runner, be it his first day or 20th year, is concerned with minutes, not miles; time, not distance. The goal is to work up to 30 minutes at a comfortable pace. The rule is to run at that comfortable pace to a point this side of fatigue.

Do not bother with distance. It is effort and time that do those good things to our bodies. This equation frees us from the tyranny of speed and distance. There is no need, then, to count laps or measure miles, no need for the stopwatch and the agonized groans that go with it. Simply dial the body to "comfortable," and go on automatic pilot. Then, continue to fatigue or 30 minutes, whichever comes first.

It is even better not to reach fatigue, but instead to come to the kitchen door or the gym still eager to do more, ready to resume on that note the next time out.

Our aim, I said, is 30 minutes. In the beginning, five minutes may be all you can handle. But quite soon—sooner, in fact, than you expect—you will be able to run continuously for 30 minutes. I have seen a 30-year-old housewife get up to 30-minute runs with a month of training and run a five-mile race within 10 weeks of buying her running shoes.

That 30 minutes is as far as we need to go. It is the endpoint of fitness. That 30 minutes will get us fit and put us in the 95 percentile for cardio-pulmonary endurance. At 12 calories per minute, it will eventually bring our weight down to desired levels. It also will slow the pulse and drop the blood pressure. It will make us good animals.

That first 30 minutes is for my body. During that half-hour, I take joy in my physical ability, the endurance and power of my running. I find it a time when I feel myself competent and in control of my body, when I can think about my problems and plan my day-to-day world. In many ways, that 30 minutes is all ego, all self. It has to do with me, the individual.

What lies beyond that fitness of muscle? I can only answer for myself. The next 30 minutes is for my soul. In it, I come upon the third-wind, which is psychological (unlike the second- wind which is physical). And then, I see myself not as an individual but as part of the universe. In it, I can happen upon anything I I ever read or saw or experienced. Every fact and instinct and emotion is unlocked and made available to me through some mysterious operation in my brain.

Recently, I came upon that feeling about 35 minutes out. I had just attacked a long hill on the river road and had been reduced to a slow jog. Then, it happened. The feelings of wholeness and peace and contentment came over me. I loved myself and the world and everything in it. I had no longer to will what I was doing. The road seemed to be running me. I was in a place and time I never wanted to leave.

To achieve fitness, there is no need to do more than 30 minutes at a comfortable pace. Past that, you must proceed with caution. Fitness can change your body. But the third wind can change your life.

HOW OFTEN?

How often must we run this 30 minutes at a comfortable pace? The answer the exercise physiologists give us is four times a week, a figure they've arrived at by testing innumerable individuals of both sexes at all ages. A four-times-a-week schedule, they assure us, will make us fit and keep us that way.

Looked at another way, this is just two hours of exercise a week. Need it be done not more than one day apart, as it is usually prescribed? Could we do all of our exercise on one day and then rest the other six? Or would it be okay to run an hour every third day and thereby satisfy the requirements?

The experts, as expected, are divided on these questions. They have not adequately explored the subject of de-training. They do not know how soon we lose the benefits of a prolonged bout of exertion. There is some reason to suspect that weekend running may be enough. I have a colleague who, for personal reasons, has limited his running to two hours or more on Saturday and a race on Sunday. On this unscientific regimen, he has broken three hours in the marathon and more often than not beats me at lesser distances.

His is just one other way to train. Training is, after all, simply a matter of applying stress, allowing the body to recover and then applying stress again. For each of us, the appropriate stress and the appropriate time to recover are different.

This is not a real problem in the minimum program of fitness. Almost anyone can handle an easy 30 minutes four times a week, an hour twice a week or even two hours once a week. But we are not minimizers; we are maximizers, and our difficulties are with doing too much rather than too little. The runner frequently gets caught up. He finds that running must be done daily, and longer and longer. The question, then, becomes not how much is *enough*, but how much is *too much*. The problem becomes not fitness but exhaustion.

All this occurs, it seems to me, because we seek not only physical fitness but psychological fitness as well. I need the minimum program for fitness because, like 95% of Americans, I have an occupation that isn't physical enough to make me fit. The 30 minutes four times a week is enough positive input to balance my negative physical output. It is not enough, however, to counteract the minuses in my day-to-day psychological life. To achieve a psychological balance, I need much more running.

How many minutes of running do I need, then, to keep in a happy frame of mind? How many times a week must I run to have a capacity for work and the ability to enjoy life?

All too often, there come days when I don't feel like running. Then, I am not sure whether I am tired or just lazy, whether I am physically exhausted or merely bored and lacking the will-power to do what I should do.

On those days when I lack zest and enthusiasm, I use the second wind to tell me whether what I'm experiencing is physical or psychological. When the second wind comes, as it does for me at the six-minute mark, I know. If the usual good feelings are there, the warm sweat and that feeling of strength and energy, I know my aversion was largely mental. I need a new route or pace or companion on the run.

If, however, I feel a cold, clammy sweat and weakness, I pack it in and go home. I have even at such times had to walk or accept a ride home, having gone less than a mile even though a few weeks before I may have run a very good marathon. Such physical exhaustion, however, is usually preceded by an elevated pulse rate in the morning. When mine is 10 beats above my usual resting pulse of 48, I know that I have once more overtrained. I need a nap instead of a workout.

So you see, it is your body that is the ultimate arbiter in your fitness program. The body tells you how fast. Dial to "comfortable," and run at a pace which would permit you to talk to a companion. The body tells you how long. Run just this side of fatigue. And the body tells you how often. Feel zest. Respond to the second wind. Note any changes in your morning pulse rate.

Follow these rules. Then, somewhere between the minimum suggested and the maximum you can handle, you will find the fitness beyond muscle that we all need to live the good life.

Chapter 5
Effects of Training

LONGER AND FASTER

Three laboratory measurements can determine if a runner is an international-class athlete: (1) rate of oxygen consumption; (2) concentration of the fatigue products lactic acid and pyruvic acid in blood plasma; (3) maximum oxygen intake.

C. H. Wyndham of South Africa used these tests to predict if a runner had the ability and training to run a sub-four-minute mile. His studies indicated that the main effect of training was on an aerobic (with oxygen) metabolic process. The maximum oxygen intake at which the lactic acid rises above normal can be raised by 10%. And the extent of the lactic acid increase at high rates of oxygen consumption is much less in the trained than in the untrained state.

Wyndham could chart no improvement in mechanical efficiency by training and found that maximum oxygen intake increased only by about 5% with training.

The main physiological characteristic of highly trained marathon runners, Wyndham said, is the ability to run for prolonged periods at 80% of maximum oxygen uptake without much evidence of anaerobic metabolism.

The South African suggested that to attain this state, men must run 20-25 miles a day at a high proportion of their maximum oxygen intake. The reason for the improvement is not clear.

Capable endurance runners are unique in their high aerobic

power-weight ratio. The average maximum oxygen intake of a 130-pound endurance runner is 27% higher than the average of fit young men of the same weight.

ANAEROBIC FITNESS

Anaerobic fitness is now the difference between winners and losers, reports physiologist Fritz Hagerman of Ohio University. Differences in aerobic capacity (maximal oxygen consumption) in top-flight runners are minimal. Races are won by fast finishes, an essentially *anaerobic* activity.

Anaerobic fitness relates to two factors: (1) lactic acid building up in the blood, and (2) use of high-energy phosphate compounds. According to Hagerman, some of this anaerobic activity goes on all the time, even in a marathon. We are not a multistage rocket shifting into another system; all systems are working simultaneously.

The best training for high-energy phosphates, he says, is 15 seconds at maximum speed with a 2-3-minute rest. This allows no significant lactic acid accumulation. The best training for lactic acid accumulation are high-intensity training runs of 220 yards to two miles. Hagerman thinks interval hill running may be the best high-intensity exercise.

FITNESS TESTING

Having an exercise physiology profile done can be even more painful psychologically than it is physically. The runner finally and irrevocably learns who he is. No longer can he regard his performances as a series of peaks and valleys leading to infinite possibilities ahead. These tests tell him what he can do and what he can't do. They also, unfortunately, tell him what he will never do and, even more unfortunately, what he should have been able to do and never did.

The runner need speculate no further on the benefits of diet and vitamins and new relaxation techniques. He now knows his limitations, what ambitions are futile and how he has wasted his talents over the years. The exercise profile is, therefore, not something to be entered into lightly. One must be ready for it.

I was. I was ready for anything Dr. David Costill and his associates at the Human Performance Laboratory at Ball State

University could tell me about myself and my body. At my age, "Know thyself" has an urgency that allows me to search for that knowledge wherever it is available, and then to make the necessary decisions and accept the consequences.

After 14 years of running with varying success at varying distances, I wanted to know just who I was. After 14 years of pursuing the goal of the three-hour marathon, I was finished with trying to be someone I was not. I had to learn whether I was really a marathoner who either didn't train enough or could not run the race with enough courage to be successful—or know for certain that I wasn't a marathoner and never would be. Whatever the answer, I was ready. I had worked on this puzzle long enough. Now, I wanted to look in the back of the book for the answer.

The maximum oxygen capacity was my first awakening. Mine was 60 which put me in the "fair" group. Those from 60-70 are defined as "good." Those above 70 are classified as "elite." Still, "fair" is not a bad classification. You can still run reasonably good times as long as you are in your correct event. And you can do even better if you have good efficiency, which is a measure of the per cent of your maximal oxygen capacity you use at submaximal effort.

My efficiency was good—in fact, 10% better than average for a group of college runners used as the standard. After these figures were in, Costill suggested that I should be able to run a 2:54 marathon. Was I, after all, just a gutless wonder who refused to discipline himself in training and had wasted the last 14 years? It seemed so, or else the three-hour mark would long ago have been achieved. The muscle biopsy would have to give me the final answer.

With the development of this biopsy technique, researchers finally reached the cellular level of the athletes where all the biochemistry takes place. And through the discovery of typical muscle patterns in champion runners, they have been able to predict performance and advise runners on their potential. From my biopsy, they would learn how much of my muscle was composed of red slow-twitch endurance fibers and how much was white fast-twitch speed fibers.

They could then match this against the figures recorded at Dallas for the country's best men distance runners, 79% slow twitch and 21% fast twitch. Distance runners are born with this slow-twitch endurance capacity and then developed by their training. This mixture is determined at birth by heredity and cannot be changd by training or anything else you may have in mind. We are born with a certain material, and then have to make the best out of what we are.

I no longer had any quarrel with this. Now, I just wanted to know. Nothing less than wanting that knowledge would have led me to lie face down on that examining table and allow Costill to introduce his outsized needle into my calf.

He had told me it would hurt less than having blood taken from my arm. He meant that to be reassuring, but I have never been one who thought having blood drawn from my arm was a minor event. I was even more disturbed when he cleared the room of some students who had newly arrived for summer work at the lab.

"They tend to faint while watching their first one," he explained.

I was beginning to have second thoughts. Perhaps I could live with that impossible 2:54 marathon ahead of me. But before I could move, Costill had struck me with the novocaine. From then on, it was routine—some pain, of course, but then the Bandaid was applied, and I was up and walking. I was also a little proud of myself and the Bandaid like some child newly out of the emergency room. I had joined the big time. I had been biopsied.

Later, Costill gave me the verdict. I had only 60% slow twitch. I was not and never would be a good marathon runner. My best race, he told me, was the two-mile. No glamour events for me. No mile or marathon. Just a race that is hard to find, difficult to train for and mean to run. You just hurt the whole last mile.

But when you go looking for the truth, you had better live with it when you find it.

MUSCLE BIOPSY

Q: Where can more information about the ratio of fast- to slow-twitch muscle fibers be found? What is a muscle biopsy, and who does one?

A: Unfortunately, this easily-done test is not generally available. Few centers in the United States do these biopsy studies. I had mine done by Dr. David Costill at the Human Performance Laboratory at Ball State University, Muncie, Ind. The test was painful, but not excessively so, and I was able to run the next day without difficulty.

Incidentally, Costill has said that a significant physical test of the fast/slow fiber ratio is the vertical jump. World-class sprinters often have a vertical jump of 30-40 inches, while milers are in the 20-30 range, and long-distance runners are usually below 20.

DAILY RUNNING

Q: I was running an average of about 6-8 miles a day, and I was feeling pretty good. But then, it became a strain to run five miles. My legs were feeling like lead, and my breathing was labored. Running is supposed to be fun, yet for me it hasn't been for a long time. Any suggestions?

A: I have found daily running to be a draining practice. I gradually use myself up and am unaware of it. A state of staleness sets in very gradually, and like most runners I try harder. The result is loss of both pleasure and ability.

I now take off at least one day every week, frequently take two days off, and more often than I would have thought possible in the past, I take three days off. If I finally become aware of and accept that I am stale, I take a nap daily instead of a run. After 3-10 days of naps, I suddenly find again that almost uncontrollable urge to run.

TRAINING TWICE DAILY

Q: I like to run from 60-90 minutes per day. My problem is that it is not always possible to have more than 30 minutes available at one time. Is it, therefore, approximately the same to run 30 minutes early in the morning and 30 later in the day as it would be to run 60 minutes at one time? Or should the pace be increased if the periods are split?

A: Splitting your running time into two sections a day theoretically provides the same fitness benefits as doing it in one session.

However, I am not quite sure this is true. In Hawaii, for instance, runners are going more and more to longer distances on an every-other-day basis.

In South Africa, where everyone seems to be in training for the 56-mile Comrades Race, the general scheme is three 8-10-milers during the week and a long, long run on Sunday—i.e., 20-30 miles.

Mostly, these distances are run at a casual pace, sometimes interspersed with stops for tea. The feeling is that a longer run every other day or every third day is worth more than splitting the weekly mileage into daily allotments.

I have switched to this type of running. My workouts are longer and longer, but I am taking more and more rest days during the week. Oddly, my mileage stays much the same.

The answer to your dilemma, then, may be the long weekend run.

MARATHON HINTS

Q: I have been running track and cross-country for four years. I want to run a marathon but am unsure of a few things. How do I train? How much distance? Speed? What type of shoes are best?

A: Marathon running is almost completely aerobic. There is no need, therefore, to train for oxygen debt and do speed work. Your entire training can be long, slow distance. This distance should be about 30 miles a week to *complete* a marathon, probaby triple that to do your best. It would be best to start with a cold-weather marathon, since 45 degrees is the optimum temperature for running distances. Hot-weather racing can be extremely taxing.

Long-distance running should be done in shoes with a relatively high heel (close to one inch), a firm heel counter, a solid shank but with good flexibility upfront, a multi-layered sole and an adequate toe box.

The best book for any would-be distance runner is Tom Osler's *Serious Runner's Handbook* (World Publications, 1978).

EASING OFF BEFORE RACES

Q: My question concerns the week preceding a marathon. Approximately how much less mileage should be performed? Is it better not to run for the preceding one or two days to rest leg muscles?

A: My own custom is to train at my regular mileage until three days before the marathon. I then take two days off so as to be ready. I have on occasion taken three days off and found that to cause psychological problems. You get to where you wonder if you can even run around the block. I am certain, however, that taking one or, better yet, two days off (or very easy) is essential to a good performance.

Each of us finds his own way. I remember seeing Bill Clark running down Boylston Street at 6 a.m. the day of the 1968 Boston Marathon and thinking to myself, he's crazy. He finished second that year.

At the 1974 race, a slight, bearded runner told me he had run three miles earlier in the morning. I said something about leaving his race back in Boston.

I didn't see him again until early that evening in an elevator at the Sheraton Hotel. Everyone was congratulating him, and only then did I realize he was winner Neil Cusack.

WARMUP

Is the warmup necessary? Indiana University researchers say "yes." A 15-minute warmup before 90-second and five-minute runs resulted in (1) higher maximum oxygen capacity; (2) lowered lactic acid; (3) higher heart rate; (4) higher muscle temperature. Warmup was at 10 kilometers per hour (about 10 minutes per mile) up a 2% grade.

TIME OF DAY

If you're looking for a personal best, compete in the evening. Studies at the Royal College of Surgeons in Ireland showed maximum performance for 30 athletes occurred between 5 p.m. and 7 p.m. All six runners tested did better in the evening than in the morning between 7 a.m. and 8 a.m.

Previous research has also suggested this. Voight, Engel and

Klein have shown a peak performance pulse index between 4 p.m. and 6 p.m. And Crockford and Davies have reported a peak between 4 p.m. and 8 p.m. in response to sub-maximal exercise on a bicycle ergometer.

AGES AND DISTANCES

Q: What distances are appropriate for junior high-aged runners (12-14) competing in school track and cross-country events?

A: Experience has shown us that 12- to 14-year-old runners can handle long-distance running, even marathon distances, without difficulty. Studies by German physiologists have shown that children at age nine have extremely favorable ratios of heart size to body weight. After reviewing available literature, a Canadian physiologist concluded that 10-year-olds are the best-conditioned people.

The major problem with young runners is the lack of experience and judgment of their coaches. Even older runners over-race, overtrain and endanger themselves. Younger runners responding to coaches rather than what their bodies tell them are particularly at hazard.

With this in mind, I suggest the following:

Racing distance is irrelevant. In fact, longer races are less demanding of the heart than shorter ones. What is essential is that the youngster has sufficient training to negotiate the distance. Training between races should total approximately 10 times the racing distance.

What this means to me is that the amount of racing should be cut down. I was against this at first, but I see that high school boys are racing three times a week in three-mile cross-country races, and are gradually getting depleted. This leads to sore throats, colds and mononucleosis.

What I'm saying is that medically there is no reason why 12-14-year-olds should not run any distance, including marathons. However, unless racing is restricted voluntarily or by rule, they are likely to develop fatigue symptoms which will have a noticeable effect on their physical and mental condition.

My suggestion is that races of two miles and less be held once or at most twice a week. Races over that distance would require longer interim training.

RUNNING AND GROWTH

Q: I am 14 and running 10-13 miles a day, with a morning and evening session. According to a recent physical I'm in perfect health, but how will running affect my growth and future health? Can I increase my mileage safely?

A: Your running should have no effect on your growth unless you try to restrict your diet and aim for some special weight. Growth corresponds to caloric intake, not to activity. Running makes for fitness, which makes for health. This also includes the concept of rest and recuperation. Your health depends on accepting stress, in your case running, and then recuperating. As long as you feel good, avoid colds and run well, you're on the right schedule.

MEN VS. WOMEN

Q: Why are women slower runners than men? Is it physical or sociological?

A: At running events involving speed or strength, women in general will definitely be slower than men. This is a physical thing, since training for such events is not nearly as important as inherent ability. However, endurance events are quite another problem. Here, the present limitations of women may be sociological. Until women get into distance running in large numbers and utilize extensive training, we cannot be sure about their capabilities.

Miki Gorman, who ran a 2:39 marathon at age 41, has certainly raised our sights on what women can do at that distance. They seem capable of doing more than they have done thus far.

WOMEN'S MUSCLES

Q: My doctor has advised me not to run because I will develop unfeminine muscles in the legs, particularly in the calves. I am very confused, because I thought that "muscle-bound" theory had been disproved.

A: The building of muscle tissue through exercise is a subject of controversy. Some types of exercises are said to build strength without bulk.

The probability is that your calves will enlarge to some extent through running, especially if you bounce while you run or get into speed work. If you develop a running style where your thighs do most of the work, this probably won't happen or will be minimal.

I recall staying at a hotel with the Russian ballet and was struck by the muscular legs of the women dancers. This suggests that jumping motions and use of the calf are instrumental in this development. I think, however, that most observers regard dancers' legs as attractive.

PART THREE:

STRESS-DEFENSE SYSTEM

"Know how to impose stress that makes you better, how to minimize or avoid stress hostile to you."

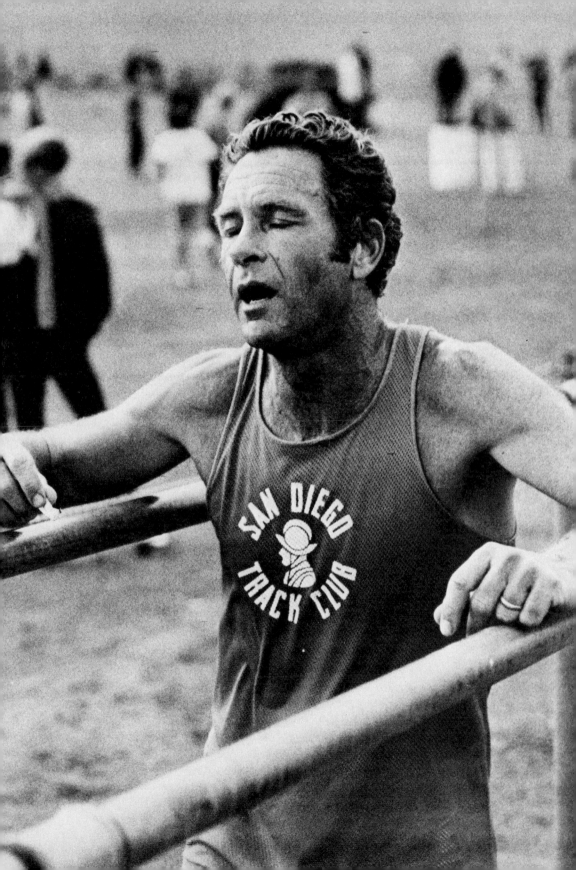

Chapter 6
The Need for Stress

Stress has been defined as any condition or situation that imposes demands for adjustment on a person. It is, therefore, a fact of life—omnipresent, inevitable. Whether it be physical, mental or emotional, it is unavoidable. And should we take to our beds and pull the covers over our heads, we simply substitute other stresses—the stress of inactivity on the body; the stress of guilt on the psyche; the stress of isolation on the mind.

Stress must be accepted, must be seen for the good it does and then managed so the bad consequences are minimized. It must be welcomed, because without it we would be less than our best.

In accepting stress, we know the truth of Nietzsche's words, "What does not destroy me makes me strong."

Stress makes us fit, ready of mind, people of virtue and courage. Stress is what makes us complete. Through it we advance, grow, stay alive. It is not without danger, of course. Stress is a struggle that can also destroy. It can weaken us physically, make us ill, cause a nervous breakdown, force us to lose faith in ourselves and creation, deliver us to the dark night of the soul.

But there is no alternative. Were I not to engage in this continuous encounter, I would give up the possibility of my development, of being stretched to my limit. I would give up all chance I have of realizing the potential I had at birth.

The business of life, then, is stress. By using instinct and intelligence, discipline and humor, a sense of play, a feeling of self-esteem, I learn to handle it.

The principles of stress and its effects are quite simple. There is the first stage of shock or alarm in which the whole force of physical and mental and psychological resources are brought to bear on the situation.

Then, in the second stage there is the gradual return to equilibrium, the restoration of the internal milieu, the process called homeostasis. The whole organism then comes to balance a notch higher than when the stress was imposed.

At times, of course, the opposite happens. The stress is too great, the time allowed for recuperation is too short, and exhaustion or breakdown occurs.

Stress can be large, small or medium. It can be physical, emotional, mental or spiritual, or combinations of any or all of these. The crisis that confronts us may be acute or lifelong. It might be a marathon or passing an examination, a domestic quarrel or a deadline on an assignment, as major as the acceptance of death or as minor as a faulty carburetor.

Each of us perceives and reacts to these stresses differently. This is as it should be. I am a unique individual. My body and mind and soul were made for me and no other. I react, if not as a unity, at least as a continuum, each of these functions in tune with the other.

My task, then, is to know myself. I must know what strengthens me and what could destroy me, how to impose stress that makes me better, how to minimize or avoid that hostile to me.

Let it be said, however, that there are no bad stresses, just as there are no bad experiences. Everything is part of the Great Experiment, part of the learning process. We learn who we are by finding the stresses that are most difficult to handle.

Chapter 7
Working Too Hard

TAKE A DAY OFF

Give Americans Wednesdays off!

That's my suggestion to the Senators who passed a billion-dollar bill intended to find a cure to the epidemic of heart disease in the United States.

Work is the cause of our heart attacks!

That's my word to the researchers who will man the 10 heart disease prevention centers and the 30 basic research centers the money will build and staff.

Forget about obesity, high cholesterol and excessive smoking. They are simply friends of the killer, incidental to the addiction Americans have for work.

Work is the real killer. It provides the stress. And coronary disease is a stress disease. Like ulcers and colitis and nervous breakdowns, it results from an overload—physical, mental, psychological or combinations of all three. The patient, in effect, blows a fuse. Work usually supplies the decisive amount of stress.

Work remains the main source of stress in a person's life (unless he has opted for the greater stress of disability, prolonged education or welfare). It also remains for most of us a satisfying and important human activity. There and there alone can many of us find creativity, self-expression, self-esteem and feelings of security. Work, said Freud, is essential to mental health. It absorbs hostility and aggression, he claimed. Work also satisfies our need to be with people, to participate and know our participation is valued, to contribute and know we are contributing.

The psychologists have told us about these good things, and I believe them. They have analyzed and reanalyzed work, looking for ways to provide involvement and satisfaction and psychological growth. They have introduced techniques to make people feel responsible and wanted and important.

But they forget one thing. We are bodies. They tend to forget about a man's guts, to ignore his heart and arteries and his colon and duodenal bulb. They need to be reminded that a man's internal milieu, that miraculous balance of water and salts and hormones, is as much at issue as his psychological adjustment.

Optimum work conditions must include an optimum work day and optimum work week. Sooner or later, physiologists will know how to measure the effects of stress on the various systems of the body. Sooner or later, we will be told the ideal work day and the ideal work week, and that it varies from person to person.

The ideal schedule, it seems to me, will have no more than two—certainly no more than three—work days in a row. There are few members of the population who can work four hard days in succession, much less five. On the fifth day, or possibly the fourth, work which exists for man's survival becomes a killer. That is the crux of the situation.

Take the athlete. He often bases his training on the hard-easy/easy-day routine. Some might run two hard days and then the easy days which may be hardly more than working up a sweat. Even ultra-long-distance runners, the 50-milers, take two days a week where they jog lightly.

The athlete knows that when stress is applied, the body must be given a chance to recoup. The worker's stress is different, but aggravation and tension and frustration add up like miles on a track. And five or four or even three of these days can be too much.

That's where Wednesday comes in—a day to adapt, a day to meditate. Sunday is for God. Saturday is for play. Wednesday is for self. Wednesday puts the rest of your week, even the rest of your life, in perspective. Used for reading, self-improvement or simply contemplating the sky, it tells you what your job really means and where it fits in the scheme of things.

The best method of coping with stress is in the rest and self-expression only Wednesday can bring: that special sanity that comes in the middle of the week when man can stand back from God and country and family and work, and for 24 hours just be himself.

SIGNS OF OVERTRAINING

Q: How can I assure myself that I'm training enough, while being careful not to do too much? It seems like a very fine line between the two.

A: Over the years, I have come to believe in two rules about training. The first, it is better to be undertrained than over-trained. The second, if things are going badly I am undoubtedly overtrained and need less work rather than more.

Is there some way to guide yourself? Yes. First, listen to your body. Second, keep a "fitness index."

The method for keeping the index is simple. When you awake in the morning, lie in bed for five minutes. Then, take

Day	Morning			Training			Post-training	
	P	W	B	M	T	S	P(immed)	P(15m)
Mon								
Tue								
Wed								
Thu								
Fri								
Sat								
Sun								

P = Pulse; W = Weight; B = Breaths/min.; M = Miles; T = Type of training, i.e. Distance, Intervals, Race; S = Speed, i.e. Easy, Moderate, Hard; If Race, insert time.

your pulse for 60 seconds. Do the same later in the day after training. Take your pulse immediately after stopping running and then 15 minutes later.

As you record these figures over the weeks, you will be able to determine your ideal figures. You must then be wary of any sudden rise in pulse rate. If the morning pulse is up 10 or more beats, you have not recovered from the previous day's training. Practice, therefore, should be limited or curtailed until the pulse returns to normal.

Q: The general indices of "overtraining" suggested by you and others are too nebulous and subjective to be of practical use. Although your system of pulse monitoring is more definitive, my post-workout readings are a function of the severity of the workout and no clear pattern emerges. Paramedical personnel conduct blood hemoglobin tests and measure blood pressure, and diabetics daily monitor their urine content. Can and should runners be trained to conduct more definitive tests of their condition to avoid overtraining?

A: Believe me, I am as upset as you are that the indices of overtraining are so imprecise. In fact, there are even some people who say no such physiological state exists—that it is all psychological.

Unfortunately, there are no definitive chemical or blood tests to indicate the onset of overtraining. The question is whether we can listen to our bodies. Some messages come through. The pulse rate, especially if followed over a prolonged period following all-out effort, is still a first-rate test.

Q: In an attempt to establish some tangible indices of overtraining, I have experimented with your suggestions of pulse reading each morning, weigh-ins and so forth. I also have noticed a pattern in my body temperature. It ranges from a morning reading of 98.2 to a late-afternoon reading of 99.4 to a late-night temperature of 97.6. What are the fluctuations showing, and what are their implications? Are these good monitors of the body's ability to handle training? Is the body best equipped to handle stresses of training at low or high temperatures?

A: The temperature cycle is one of our circadian rhythms, and one of the most stable. Abnormalities have been reported in certain sleep disturbances, where the temperature continues to rise during the night.

What you are reporting is the normal cycle. The absolute levels could be of interest, but they do fluctuate with environmental temperature, so interpretation would have to be guarded.

CHRONIC FATIGUE

Q: I am sluggish and weak in my training runs, and fatigue lingers. I've noticed that my glands are swollen at certain times and that I have trouble with allergies. I have had this problem for several months. Could this be a low-grade infection, and what can be done to correct it?

A: Chronic fatigue is a difficult problem to handle. The most obvious answer is that a runner would be overtraining. Lack of zest for practice is a sign to do slow work and to rest alternate days until you get the old desire back.

In overtrained athletes, allergies tend to get worse, and glandular enlargement sometimes occurs. Insomnia, poor attention span, weight loss, rash and a variety of other symptoms can occur. Rest is the only remedy.

On the other hand, you may have had infectious mononucleosis and not allowed yourself sufficient rest to spring back. Again, allergies would be prominent. I doubt that you have a low-grade infection.

The amount of work each runner can handle (especially speed work) is highly individual. You must set up your own distance program, and use swollen glands and increased allergies as indications that you have pushed too hard.

UPS AND DOWNS

Q: I suffer from a running "yo-yo syndrome." The cycle starts with a steady progress which lasts from a few weeks to a few months. Then, for no apparent reason, my condition starts to degenerate. When I am at the top of the yo-yo, my resting pulse rate is 65. When I'm at the bottom, the pulse is 75.

A: You are experiencing cycles that affect every runner. There are several peaks during the year that are maintained for 6-10 weeks. Then, the runner should back off for a few weeks.

If you don't you will have to suffer through a prolonged, severe exhaustion. Accept those rhythms which you cannot alter. No human, no animal, improves in a straight line. We plateau out, then dip down before we progress again.

As you have already noted, your resting pulse gives the game away. When you get that 10-point rise, you should take a nap instead of a four-mile run. Learn to do that; learn to listen to your body.

TRAINING IS A STRESS

Q: I am interested in training procedures which provide the greatest improvement for the least amount of effort. Do you have some suggestions?

A: Training has a simple formula: Stress is applied, followed by a rest period during which the body returns to equilibrium at a somewhat higher level of fitness.

This can be a highly individualized response. Aerobic training may be done best by increasing both the total load and the rest time, say by taking just two very long runs a week. Faster training might be done also by taking a single short, hard run (say 600 yards) each day.

SLEEP

Q: I've been told that the healthier you are, the less sleep you need. Does that mean a person could cut down on the amount of sleep needed by running more (this would be after he gets into better condition from the extra running, of course)?

A: You've been told incorrectly. Lack of necessary sleep is one of the major faults in training. When in heavy training, the runner needs more, not less sleep.

Jim Councilman of Indiana has his swimmers sleeping nine hours a night plus a nap in the afternoon when they are in heavy training. I doubt that runners are some special breed that can do without sleep.

Sleep is an active process during which some body functions actually reach their peak. Research has shown that sleep replenishes certain essential substances in the brain. Depletion of these substances seems to have a causal relation with depressive states. Sleep is also a major factor in the secretion of growth hormones.

It could be that sleep is the one factor not sufficiently emphasized in training.

Q: I readily agree with you about the need for extra sleep. But I think the paradox of being restless—or simply not tired—with increased running needs to be explained. Personally, after several months of moderate running, I begin to have difficulties sleeping. Eventually, I feel I am "speeding"—i.e., I feel full of energy, but I also become frenetic, "hyper." A few days rest is always a solution, but I can too easily find excuses to run.

A: When a runner overtrains, he frequently develops "depression insomnia." He gets to sleep easily, but wakes up repeatedly during the night for no good reason and frequently has trouble getting back to sleep.

This happens to me when I overrace or do excessive speed work. I use it as a sign that I am going past my peak, and I cut back on training and competition.

I, therefore, do not consider this decreasing need for sleep as a normal physiological state. If so, it would be accompanied by better and better performances. In fact, it is usually accompanied by a deterioration in my times as well as my general physical state.

In many ways, this sleep pattern is the most sensitive indicator of an approaching exhaustion state. It should be brought to the attention of both runners and coaches.

Chapter 8
Results of Excess Stress

MONO

When Prince Albert died of typhoid, the disgruntled British press—according to Dr. Alex Comfort, the expert on aging—referred to medicine as "the withered arm of science."

If that attitude is still prevalent among the general populace, one of the reasons is infectious mononucleosis—the "kissing disease." This disease continues to stump the experts while it hits the healthiest segment of our population, the young adults—and the healthiest segment of that group, the young athletes.

The boys in the white lab coats are getting desperate. They have been unable to satisfy the rules of their own infection game, rules known as Koch's postulates: (1) find the bug; (2) give the bug to a volunteer who gets the disease; (3) retrieve the bug.

They have a prime suspect in the bug department called the EB virus. But they can't get past Step Two. Not even kissing will give it to a volunteer. My guess is that nothing will until they move their experiments out to the athletic field. They may have the right virus, but what they don't have is exhaustion.

Exhaustion is the key. Mono may be a virus disease. ("I am of the opinion," writes Dr. Betty Jo White in *Infectious Diseases*, "that the patient has the virus in him forever.") It may even be an autoimmune disease where the patient reacts to his own body as suggested by the late hematologist William

Dameshek. But it rarely exists and almost never recurs without exhaustion.

Coaches are proving that every day. Wherever you find a team heading for regional or national ranking, you are likely to find mononucleosis hitting the stragglers. Wherever you find champions on a squad, you are likely to find others in the infirmary.

Coaches must learn to individualize (and runners who coach themselves must learn to coach *themselves*—not some ideal runner their age) about hard work.

Hard work is not always bad. Some runners can accept it and become champions. Other would-be champions are destroyed by it. The coach who lumps his athletes together and gives uniform workouts will prove Darwin's "survival of the fittest" and wreck his team.

What happens may be called mononucleosis. Some call it staleness. Some call it "peaking too soon." But the symptoms are the same, and so are the effects: fatigue, swollen glands, poor attention span, restless sleep, bad performances. The bad performances are characteristic. The runner may suspect all is not right, but the initial part of the race holds no hint of disaster. Only in the last fourth of the race, as Yale Coach Bob Giegengack observed, does the runner come apart. When he reaches back for the final lift, he finds he has nothing left.

Mono symptoms range from failure only under race conditions to an acute febrile illness with such problems as sore throat, tonsillitis, loss of appetite, jaundice, rash and joint pains. Such an episode may also have occurred in the runner's past, with or without confirmation in a "mono-test."

Some physicians claim one attack gives you a lifelong immunity against catching the disease again. If so, runners are not getting new attacks but relapses of their old disease. It is true that when symptoms return (usually in milder form), the "mono-test" is not positive. But runners certainly recognize their state as similar in kind, if not degree, to the mono attack.

Perhaps all we can say is that exhaustion in a certain group of individuals can cause a "mono-like" state. The treatment is rest, then every-other-day easy workouts until zest and the desire to train are regained—and workouts again become enjoyable. The temptation to race and find out if one is well again should be resisted as long as possible.

Reduced activity and tincture of time are the essentials in the treatment of this disease.

FLU

Pride goeth before the flu.

In Seaside, Ore., I had run my fastest marathon of my career, an amazing (to me) 3:01:25. It was a race I had started with every intention of simply making a fair showing, a nice respectable time for my hosts who had been good enough to ask me out to speak the night before the race.

But as the early miles passed, I began to feel better and better. My concern over using up too much strength and energy before the annual visit to Boston began to fade.

I had begun to knock off consecutive seven-minute miles, a pace that would bring me in around 3:04, when it suddenly struck me I had a chance to get in under the magical three-hour limit that had always eluded me.

When I still felt strong at the 18-mile mark, I said to myself, "To hell with Boston," and began to cut loose. By 20 miles, I was under seven-minute pace and reaching for the 6:52 average that would put me under three hours.

It was not to be. I had given away too much time in the first miles, but still it was the best I had ever done. I was clearly in the best shape of my life.

Back home, I started on speed work to sharpen for the Eastern Masters Championships. But something seemed wrong. Everything seemed to be a great effort.

Then, the flu struck. The influenza virus is a submicroscopic particle. How it accomplishes its ravages is beyond me. My flu started with a sore throat and then progressed to a cough. At one point, I thought my lungs would come out inverted like an umbrella on a windy day.

The fever came and with it went all interest in anything but survival. I finally went to bed for two days, the first medical problem to put me there since I had hepatitis 25 years ago.

The weakness persisted. Only much later did I face the day with any curiosity about what is going to happen, with any zest in living. Running was out of the question until the bug let me out of its grip.

Even the virologists are in doubt as to why the bug has such a grip. Apparently, the virus somehow gets into the cells, reproduces itself and attacks the membrane or outer lining of the cell, finally killing it and moving on to attack another cell.

Why this makes you feel as if someone has plugged in to your energy source and siphoned it all out, I'm not sure. What it does is bring you up short on the old agenda game.

Agenda is simply the what-I'm-going-to-do-tomorrow-and-the-next-day-and-the-next, the how-great-I'm-going-to-be-in-the-future. Flu changes all that. It brings you back to now and makes you thankful for the basics. Being alive, for instance, and having available to you enough strength to start all over again, just as if it were the first day you bought your running shoes.

When you come back, it is difficult at times to know whether fatigue is physical or psychological. There is, however, a simple test for this. Start your runs very slowly until you reach the point where you start to sweat. This usually takes about six minutes. At this point, you should feel like running no matter how you felt in the beginning. If you don't and five more minutes confirms it, pack it in. Throw away your agenda for today.

When you throw away the agenda, you taste the food you are eating right now instead of thinking about dessert. And you begin to hear what your body is telling you this instant instead of dreaming of glory and perfection. Pride is nothing more than looking beyond the present moment.

I'm glad I had that marathon. But I won't be too broken up if I never have another like it or go under three hours. All I want is to be myself in health and enjoy today. Tomorrow and Boston can take care of themselves.

Q: I came down with the flu, which lasted about three days but left me weak. I'm wondering how long a runner should wait before resuming training after a bout with the flu.

A: The rule of thumb in an illness like the flu is to expect to feel poorly for the period of fever and then to have a convalescence twice as long as the feverish period.

If the fever takes five days, then an additional ten days might be needed before you feel nearly normal. Short of that length of time, you should train gingerly with attention to fatigue and possible relapse.

Running with a fever and a flu can be dangerous. Sudden death can occur if the virus is also affecting the heart muscle, which it frequently does.

COLDS

Q: What do you recommend when I have a cold, sore throat or am not feeling up to par: (a) stop completely until all symptoms are gone; (b) moderate running, but do not stop completely; (c) continue normal running no matter how I feel?

A: I treat colds with respect. It is my feeling that they represent a breakdown of the defense system. The cold is an early warning of exhaustion. Because of this philosophy, I tend to draw back on my training.

Depending on the symptoms, I may stop running for one to three days and then resume a slow pace for relatively short distances. However, I do not wait for all the symptoms to subside unless there seems to be a major bronchial element in the infection. I do think that the sore throat should clear before you do any serious running.

Q: For the past few years, I have noticed that I get a cold just after a race for which I've done excessive exertion. I get two or three a year, usually following a big race. What do you suggest?

A: The common cold is the most frequent overuse illness in runners. We do not catch colds; we run ourselves into them.

I do just that three or four times a year. Just when I am peaking out, having my best times, hearing tunes of glory, I wake up with a scratchy throat. It usually takes 7-10 days to right things.

Mostly, as you say, it follows an exceptionally good performance. It's the old story—when you are at your peak, you are a razor's edge from disaster.

The answer, it seems to me, is to peak only a few times a year, for races that have tradition and meaning. Otherwise, it is best to monitor your waking pulse and back off when it rises to

10 beats above normal.

SWOLLEN GLANDS

Q: I am an active road runner and over the last five months have noticed symptoms that my family doctor cannot explain, namely extensive swollen lymph glands.

When I first noticed the swollen nodes (after a hard half-marathon), there were many in the groin area but only one was sore. Later, I noticed a swollen node on my neck and some small ones in my armpits. I think the neck swelling is more noticeable when I am training hard (more than 70 miles a week) and losing weight. After races, when I relax a little and eat more, the swelling subsides and the slight discomfort disappears altogether.

Since I continue to run well and feel healthy, my doctor feels the symptoms are running-related. I tend to agree, but if you could provide an explanation, I would be most grateful.

A: Lymph glands do enlarge in periods of overstress. Enlarged lymph glands are, in fact, one of the signs seen in staleness. These glands do not, however, get to be any size, and they do subside when the exhaustion passes.

It seems to me that your physician is taking the sensible approach. He has, after all, palpated innumerable lymph nodes, and these just do not impress him.

Usually, biopsy of groin glands is unrewarding, and your others don't seem of a size to be pathological. Further studies could be done to see if you have any nodes inside, but, personally, I'd forget it. I think 70 miles a week would make my lymph glands swell.

PART FOUR:
MUSCULOSKELETAL SYSTEM

*"You must listen to your body.
Run through annoyance but not through pain."*

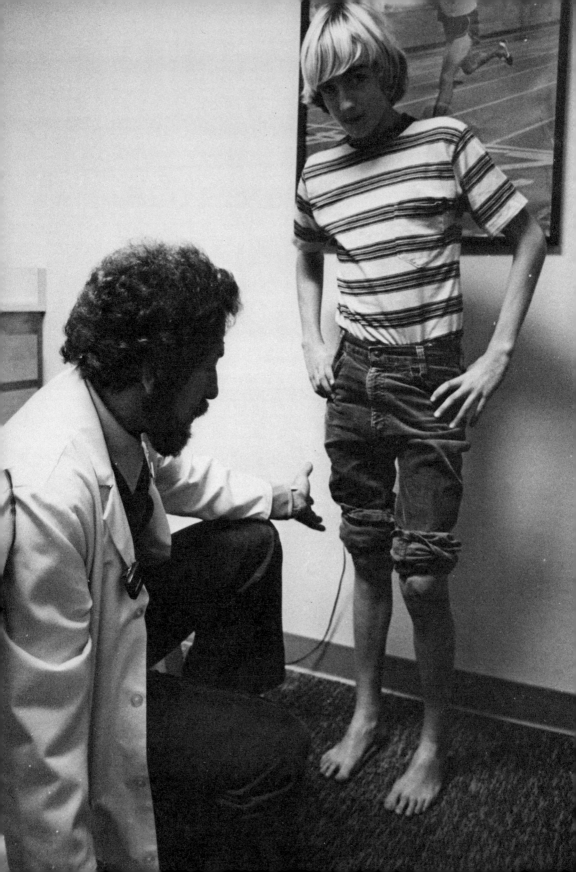

Chapter 9
Structural Weaknesses

When I began running back in the early 1960s, I did not realize that treatment of the runner was still in its medical infancy. It was some time before I recognized the void existing in the diagnosis and treatment of overuse syndromes of the lower extremity and low back.

At that time, there was a vacuum in the area between the family physician and the field of orthopedic medicine. And, unfortunately, it was just that specialty or group of specialties in between that was needed to keep the runner running—not only running but running pain-free.

The story of the evolution of medical care for musculo-skeletal disease of the lower extremity is the story of orthopedic medicine and of the two major advances in sports medicine in the last decade. They are (1) sports podiatry, the diagnosis and treatment of foot conditions as they relate to overuse problems in the lower extremity and low back; (2) muscle strength/flexibility balance—the effect of imbalance both locally, on the muscles themselves, and on the functions of the foot and other joints.

During the past decade, we have come to understand that certain foot types predispose the runner to injury. Dudley Morton's discovery of the "atavistic" foot, the foot with the short big toe and long second toe, has been resurrected. Once again, we are aware that such feet have a laxity along the inner border from heel to big toe which allows excessive pronation during footstrike.

This hypermobile foot and excessive pronation have now been implicated in numerous overuse syndromes of the foot, leg, knee, thigh and low back. This genetically inferior foot occurs in about one-third of the population and is probably a major factor in running injuries.

Less common but more difficult to treat is the second type of biomechanically weak foot, the "pes cavus" or high-arched foot. This occurs in 5-10% of the population but is seen with much greater frequency in doctors' offices. The sports podiatrists I have talked to say that as much as 30-40% of their patient load is due to the high-arched foot.

This foot, instead of being hypermobile, is too rigid. Where the hypermobile foot needs control and will respond to almost anything stuffed into a shoe, the high-arched foot needs movement to absorb shock. Therefore, a "control" shoe which will help a Morton's foot may immediately give symptoms in a high-arched foot.

In the beginning, in that first burst of enthusiasm, we thought sports podiatry could do it all. Just have the appropriate support made, and all would be well. It didn't work that way. Orthotics failed, and failed for a number of reasons. Some were casted wrong. Others over- or undercorrected. Still others were not adjusted in followup visits. But by far the most failed because there were other factors that put too much stress on the functioning foot. These were muscle strength/flexibility imbalance, shoes and surfaces.

The case for muscle flexibility to prevent muscular injuries was first made by Paul Uram, a gymnastics coach from Butler, Pa., who is now the "flex" coach of the Pittsburgh Steelers. Before Uram, most athletes thought weight training was the way to injury prevention. Uram saw from his work in gymnastics that this was incorrect. What was needed was balance—both strength and flexibility.

His ideas worked in football and now they are working in running. What we came to find out was that when a runner trains, three things happen to the muscles and two are bad. The prime-movers, the actual propulsion muscles, become strong, tight and inflexible. The antagonists, the opposite muscles that control the action, become relatively weak.

The effects of these imbalances are twofold. First, such an imbalance feeds down to the footstrike, preventing the leg from coming over and past the foot at plant. The needed 10-15 degrees past perpendicular is absorbed into an already pronating arch or creates increased shock in the rigid foot. Secondly, imbalances between shin and calf lead to shin splints, just as imbalance of quads and hamstrings leads to pulls, and imbalances between low back and belly muscles lead to sciatica, or low-back pain.

The knowledge of appropriate inserts for the shoes and sufficient exercising for muscle strength/flexibility imbalance should have been enough, but it wasn't. The shoes and surfaces also entered into the production of injuries in runners.

We have seen especially over the last few years a proliferation of apparent improvement in shoes. Unfortunately, what has happened has been a tradeoff. Whenever a shoe became better for a hypermobile foot, it almost automatically became bad for a rigid foot. The wide flanged heels which did well for the Morton's foot caused havoc in a pes cavus. Then, too, the runner with shin splints found a good deal of rubber under the ball of the foot helped, but the resultant inflexibility caused grief to the Achilles. Some runners discovered that at times a tennis sneaker would take them farther than the number-one shoe in the experts' polls. Others have successfully used garage mechanic shoes, Hush Puppies, ordinary street shoes and even bedroom slippers.

We discovered early on that the slant of the road contributed to foot and leg problems. Running against traffic caused the uppermost foot on the crest to pronate and thereby have more symptoms. Switching to the other side was helpful but proved to be too dangerous for real consideration. Also, running on pavement, which seems to bother some runners not at all, proved to be quite stressful for those with the pes cavus. They found dirt and grass much more suitable.

Finally, it became apparent both from personal experience and from polls of the runners that racing and hill work were also productive of injury. Mileage had a break-even point of about 25 miles per week, after that injuries increased almost arithmetically with mileage so that at 50 miles a week injuries were doubled.

It has been my feeling that some of this increased difficulty in racing may be due to wearing racing shoes which are in most cases little more than gloves. Wearing training shoes in races seems the best thing to do. Oddly, they may even give better performance due to better shock absorption.

As sports medicine developed, we came more and more to look at the foot, to encourage the use of stretching and strengthening exercises and to the wearing of the best shoes for each particular type of foot. Finally, we came to see that while most problems of the foot and knee could be controlled by these measures, those from the knee up often had other factors present.

In injuries involving the thigh, hip and low back, two additional elements were frequently present. The first was leg-length discrepancy or lateral asymmetry. This often was found in intractable conditions involving hip and groin and sciatic pain. The second was minor abnormalities of the lumbosacral spine, usually thought to be of no clinical significance.

What actually happens is that these minor deviations are made major by the introduction of the second element, an imbalance between the low-back muscles and the belly muscles. This combination makes the low back symptomatic. Similarly, the hip can hurt, or groin problems can develop. In both of these, muscle tightness and/or weakness are major causative factors.

When faced with an overuse syndrome, no matter what its nature, the runner must do a systems analysis which involves:

1. *Foot.* Is it a Morton's foot or a high-arched "cavus" foot? Does it demonstrate some telltale signs of failing? These are calluses under the second or third metatarsals, a heel bump on the outside upper edge, the big toe pointing toward the little toe or flat feet. If any of these are present, they probably contribute to the injury no matter where it is.

2. *Strength/flexibility.* Can you touch your fingers to your toes and hold for 60 seconds? Can you flex your foot on your ankle through 10 degrees of motion? Can you lie on your back and, holding the knees locked, touch the floor behind you with your toes? Are your leg, thigh and low-back muscle ratios all in

balance for front and back strength?

3. *Leg length.* Is one leg longer than the other? If so, how does your back compensate?

4. *Shoes.* Are you wearing a "control" shoe or a "shock-absorbing" shoe? Are your heels too wide? Too low? Is there too little rubber upfront? Too much? Do you have enough room for your toes? Is there enough control in the heel counter? Have you recently changed shoes? Let your present shoes wear down too much?

5. *Form.* Are you overstriding, reaching out, making excessive noise? Are you landing properly, with the knee bent and the foot never getting in front of the knee? Are you using your upper body for balance, as you should?

6. *Surface.* Are you allowing for the slant of the road? The slant of the beach? The turns on the track (particularly the indoor track with its tight turns)?

All of these areas can be causes of injury. I discovered many of them over the years, and I discovered at the same time to stay away from doctors. Mostly, they would warn me against continuing to run and never seemed to give me anything constructive to do. Even in this enlightened age, it is probably best for the runner to try to handle as much of the problem as possible before seeking medical help. To this end, a number of things can be done. Some involve immediate treatment, others are longterm measures aimed at prevention of injury.

Your feet, leg length and low-back abnormalities were given to you at birth. They are God's fault, so there is nothing much you can do about them. What you have to do is adjust to them, offer the body some support.

When symptoms related to a failing foot occur, there is generally a need for a controlling device. The best thing to start with is an over-the-counter arch support. The Flexos made by Dr. Scholl's are to me insubstantial but occasionally are of great benefit. Should they fail, you can try Dr. Scholl's "610s" or "Athletic A."

For leg-length problems, a simple heel lift may work. This is put in the shoe on the short-leg side. There is also value in wearing a back support when you have sciatic pain.

Supports for the knee and ankle are sometimes helpful for a number of problems. Elastic braces offer stability to the injured area.

Of course, these measures are only the beginning. If a muscle imbalance exists, it is your fault, and it is your job to reestablish that balance. Stretching and strengthening must be daily procedures. Ballet dancers do as much as 45 minutes of warming up daily, while runners do less than 10% that much. Unfortunately, it shows.

The choice of shoes comes next. In general, the narrower the heel the better for the high-arched foot; the wider the heel the better for the Morton's foot. High-arched runners generally need shoes with more shock absorption; "Morton's" runners need more control.

Whenever injury strikes, especially after months of troublefree running, you must think of what has changed. Have you suddenly increased your mileage? Gone for a long run or race in a different brand of shoes? Begun to do hill or speed work? Changed surfaces? Stopped doing your exercises? Or failed to increase your exercises as you increased your mileage? Have you switched from a track to roads or vice versa?

You must be constantly aware of causes and effects when your health is at stake.

Chapter 10
Look First at Feet

FOOT FAULTS

Today, I logged another hour of pain-free running on the roads. I am no longer bothered with metatarsal pain, plantar fascitis, heels spurs, Achilles tendinitis, shin splints, posterior tibial tendinitis or chondromalacia of my knee. Despite my 5000 footstrikes on each foot every hour, these overuse injuries should never return.

The reason? I have learned about the foot. I know now that the foot can cause pain anywhere from the big toe to the buttocks. And I know it is the inadequate, unstable, architecturally defective foot which causes most of these running woes. I have discovered five ways to finger this failing foot.

I was completely ignorant of this in my running beginnings. I had been a doctor before I became a distance runner, but that was no help. I had been taught nothing pertaining to the moving foot. In the anatomy lab, the foot was immobile and non-weight-bearing. And even at this date, the function and physiology of this 26-bone structure are difficult for me to comprehend.

I have not even an inkling of the physics of the foot. I don't understand how it goes from being a loose adaptor to a rigid lever. I know practically nothing about what happens during footstrike, midstance and toeoff in the running foot, and even less of the biomechanical evaluation of the foot at rest.

Because of this, I am unable to diagnose the myriad of structural defects in the foot which are visible only to the experts. Nor can I explain why these deficiencies result in injuries to the foot itself, the guy ropes that support it, and even the bones and joints quite distant from it.

Nevertheless, I can now recognize a foot which makes you susceptible to these things. A little knowledge may be danger- ous, but not if it gets you to someone who has a lot of it, not if it gets you to someone whose day is filled with observing and thinking about the foot and its difficulties, not if you arrive at a foot specialist with a special interest in athletes, the sports podiatrist.

If you are having pains anywhere in your feet or legs, take off your shoes and look for these telltale findings:

FOOT FAULTS

Morton's Foot   Hagland Bump   Halux Valgus

Flat Foot   Callus

1. *Morton's foot.* The Grecian foot with the short big toe and the long second; the big toe segment is short and loose so the inner border of the foot does not bear weight until late in the foot cycle. This allows the foot to flatten and pronate (tip over on the inside). Result? Any or all of the overuse syndromes runners experience.

2. *Pronation.* First, observe the arch in your foot while it is held in the air. Now, stand on both feet with the feet in the usual angle of footplant during walking or running, See if the arch flattens and the foot tips so the inner ankle bone becomes more prominent and the heel tilts inward. This action with every footstrike creates havoc with the foot-leg continuum. You can now see why drugs, cortisone shots and whirlpool are of no value. What you need, of course, is a support to prevent this when you get back on the road (an arch support that will hold your foot in that neutral non-weight-bearing position from footstrike to toeoff).

3. *Hagland's deformity.* This is a bump on the upper and outer aspect of the heel bone, caused by an abnormal movement of the heel with each footstrike.

4. *Hallux valgus.* The big toe, instead of pointing forward, begins to point toward the outside of the foot, another sign of adjustments being made to faulty biomechanics in the foot and additional evidence of a vulnerable defective foot.

5. *Callus formation.* Callus on the ball of the foot under the second or third metatarsal head is another proof of incorrect weight-bearing. It is confirmation that the area is subject to disproportionate stress. When present, it means that there is an asymmetry in the footstrike and consequent origin of an abnormal kinetic chain reaction. Callus means that evil forces are at work.

6. *High-arched foot.* This is the "pes cavus," the foot with a high instep. It has a relatively small weight-bearing area and is usually associated with very tight calf muscles. This is a rigid foot and does not move enough. Because of all these features, it accepts shock poorly.

FOOT PHYSICS

The new sports medicine is sports physics. The new sports injuries are the overuse syndromes, the biomechanical effects of excessive training on a susceptible individual. The new sports therapies are, therefore, directed at reestablishing postural and structural balance. And the new sports research is the investigation of abnormal forces acting in and on the foot, leg, knee and low back. It starts with trigonometry and ends in the mechanics of structure.

The new sports medicine is no longer concerned with drugs or surgery or acupuncture or whirlpool baths. This new sports medicine is occupied with engineering phenomena like torque and stress and strain and faulty vectors. The new sports medicine has deserted witchcraft and finally turned to science.

This scientific analysis has disclosed that our overuse syndromes have two basic causes. One is postural, the other structural.

The structural factor is a skeletal tendency, an affliction we were born with. The most frequent is what Dudley Morton in his classic *The Human Foot* called a "continuance of the pre-human condition" or more simply an atavistic foot. Such a foot still has qualities suitable for climbing trees. The big toe still has thumblike characteristics, and there is a looseness along the inner border from heel to the big toe.

The most atavistic foot is the one that has come to be called Morton's foot.

MORTON'S FOOT

The cause of *all* foot ailments, according to Dr. Dudley Morton, is faulty weight-bearing on the first metatarsal head. This coupled with a tight calf muscle is the basis of all disabling foot conditions.

Q: What abnormalities of the foot are associated with faulty weight-bearing on the first metatarsal head?

A: Morton described three conditions: The first, now called Morton's foot, is quite visible. It is the short big toe/long second toe that marks the *short first metatarsal bone*.

The other two are diagnosed by x-ray or expert examination: The loose or *hypermobile first metatarsal*; and the posterior or *backward-placed sesamoids* (little bones under the metatarsal heads) which provide the striking area.

Q: What is the common disturbance in weight-bearing in these three conditions?

A: In Morton's foot, the five metatarsal heads share the weight unevenly. The second takes the bulk of the weight. The first not only fails to take its share, but takes it too late and the foot pronates or rolls over to the inside. The tight calf cord puts even greater pressure on this area.

Q: If Morton's foot is potentially harmful, why is it so prevalent in the normal population?

A: Morton's foot (visible) occurs in about 33% of the general population. However, in a patient population of 1000 studied by Dr. Richard Schuster, 80% of the patients had the short first toe/long second configuration. No x-ray studies were done to determine how many of the other 20% had the occult forms of Morton's foot. Probably all of them did.

Q: Why is Morton's foot particularly bad in athletics?

A: The enormous amount of training puts great stress on this abnormal weight-bearing mechanism. The distance runner averages 5000 footstrikes per foot during each hour of practice. The tennis, basketball, volleyball or soccer player probably does almost as much.

In addition, the training of the runner tends to tighten the calf and thigh muscle, putting even greater stress on an already overloaded architectural error.

Q: Do we have any definite scientific evidence that Morton's foot causes foot disorders?

A: The most clearcut evidence is in the case of stress fractures of the second metatarsal bone. This fracture is quite frequent on foot soldiers and runners. It is one of the many overuse syndromes that puzzle sports physicians. If Morton is right, stress fractures should be due to overloading the second metatarsal and, therefore, should occur specifically in people with Morton's foot. This appears to be the case.

I recently surveyed all the available x-ray and orthopedic texts in the local hospital, and discovered that *every* stress fracture in these books had occurred in a Morton's foot!

Q: Is there any other way to prove that there is abnormal weight-bearing on the second metatarsal head in Morton's foot and the disorders secondary to it?

A: Yes, by Wolff's Law. This states that every change in the function of a bone is followed by a certain definite change in its internal architecture and alterations in its external configuration. X-rays of Morton's foot show just such changes in the second metatarsal. It becomes larger and wider.

Q: What disorders of the foot are associated with Morton's foot?

A: Stress fractures of the metatarsals, plantar fascitis, heel spurs and arch pain, among others.

Q: Can Achilles tendinitis occur with Morton's foot?

A: Of course, the improper weight-bearing eventually results in stretching of the arch and instability of the heel. This minute but significant tipping-over movement with each footstrike pulls on the Achilles and irritates it.

Q: What other leg conditions can result from Morton's foot?

A: Practically all the overuse syndromes of the leg, including stress fractures of the fibula and posterior tibial tendinitis, are secondary to the pronatory (tipping over inside) movement allowed by the faulty weight-bearing of that first metatarsal.

Q: What about knee pain?

A: This is almost always due to this abnormal pronation which occurs with the Morton's foot. The way to treat leg and knee troubles is to ignore them and attend to the Morton's foot.

Q: How should one go about treating a Morton's foot?

A: First, it is necessary to establish the diagnosis. Usually, the Morton's foot is visible. If the foot appears normal, it would best to x-ray it. This will establish: whether you have a hypermobile first metatarsal or posterior-placed sesamoid; whether or not the second metatarsal is hypertrophied (enlarged),

thereby establishing the presence of significant abnormal
weight bearing.

Q: Once the diagnosis is made, what treatment is available?

A: Dudley Morton suggested that the patient use a platform
of felt or inner sole under the first metatarsal area. This is still
the mainstay of treatment. But by the time the athlete is symptomatic, many secondary changes in the foot have taken place.
Therefore, a full foot orthotic (support), preferably soft or
non-rigid, may be needed. The minimum treatment, it seems to
me, would be a heel stabilizer (or a shoe with a good counter)
plus a longitudinal arch and a metatarsal extension.

The effect of the tight calf muscle should not be underestimated. Flexibility exercises may hold the key to cure, even with
the best of foot care.

THE HIGH ARCH

If you are a distance runner, your chances of developing an
overuse syndrome of the foot, leg, knee, hip or low back depend
primarily on the type of foot you have. Mileage, racing, hill
work and strength/flexibility imbalance make major contributions, of course. But the most important variable in the injury
equation is whether or not you have a biomechanically weak
foot, and if so what kind: the well-known Morton's foot with its
short big toe and long second toe, or the hitherto ignored high-
arched foot, known in medical circles as a pes cavus.

The high-arched foot is a more subtle killer. Where the Morton's foot moves too much, the cavus foot moves too little. It is
not hypermobile; it is rigid. And this rigidity renders it unable
to absorb shock. Movement is necessary to dissipate shock, and
this foot will not move. It comes down "clunk," and the impact
is transmitted directly back into the foot and up the outer side
of the leg and knee and hip.

This difficulty in handling shock is compounded by other
features of the high-arched foot. Everything about it is short
and tight. The toes tend to claw. The plantar fascia which runs
from toe to heel is decreased. The calf muscle is invariably short
and inflexible. Everything tends to diminish the weight-bearing
area and limit motion, thereby accentuating the bad effects of

the forces on the foot as it contacts the ground.

The Morton's foot is easy to treat. Its movement must be diminished, and almost anything put in the shoe will help. Once, when I was in Seattle without my arch supports, I used a folded wine list from the bedside table in my hotel room and ran without difficulty.

The problem with the high-arched foot is the opposite. The task with it is to avoid too much control, to avoid restriction. Otherwise, you get into the injuries usually associated with the cavus foot. The cavus foot, you see, is already too restricted. It cannot tolerate any further control. What it needs is more movement rather than less.

The shoe requirements for these two types of feet are, therefore, diametrically opposed. When runners wonder why their friends' supershoes are duds for them, they should compare feet.

The basic shoe for a Morton's foot is a control shoe with a good, solid, wide heel and some flexibility but little compressibility in the sole. The high-arched foot, on the other hand, needs shock absorption, with the highest heel available and good flexibility. But most of all, it cannot be restricted.

I know of one runner with a cavus foot who was running six miles a day in tennis sneakers with no trouble. He was induced by a friend to change to a top running shoe and immediately developed lateral knee pain. Such incidents are common. Shoes that are excellent for one type of foot are a disaster for another. Then, too, the number-one shoe is judged on so many factors that it is like a decathlon star—fairly good at everything and excellent at nothing.

The difficulty with the cavus foot is now being reflected in the patient load of the sports podiatrists. While it occurs in approximately 5% of the population (for comparison, the Morton's foot occurs in 33%), it is present in as many as 30-40% of runners seeking aid from those specialists.

What, then, can be done about the high-arched foot?

The answer, as I have already pointed out, is to do everything you can to diminish the effect of shock impact. This can be done in several ways, and in most instances all of them may be necessary.

1. *Shoes.* These should have good shock absorption, especially in the heel. The heel should be high, the ball of the foot wide, and there should be a sizable toe box. Racing should always be done in these training shoes.

2. *Exercises.* The cavus foot victim must be a lifetime exerciser. Daily stretching is essential in the struggle against injury. A tight calf is an invitation to injury.

3. *Orthotics.* These devices increase the weight-bearing area of the foot. This is essential because the cavus foot uses only about 35% of the foot surface. The orthotic should also function to absorb shock and prevent any abnormal motion. Appropriate materials must be used.

4. *Running form.* Shock impact is reduced by shortening the stride and reducing the noise in running. Overstriding and slapping down contribute to shock and symptoms.

The main thing is not to give up. You come from a breed that crossed continents on foot, whether Morton's or high-arched. Ten miles a day should be no problem.

SHORT LEG

Q: You have mentioned the short-leg syndrome but never fully explained it. Just what is it?

A: The short-leg syndrome refers to those foot, leg, knee and low-back problems that are caused by one leg being shorter than the other.

Usually, the dominant leg is the longer. People are right-legged and left-legged just as they are right- and left-handed. Frequently, the shortening is only from the ankle down and caused by weakness in the foot.

Correction through heel lift and/or an arch support will, in many instances, give quite astonishing relief of long-standing aches and pains. Oddly enough, the symptoms are frequently in the longer rather than the shorter leg.

Q: I recently found out through x-rays of my pelvis that my left leg is exactly one inch longer than my right leg. Is such a significant different in leg length very rare, and how severely does it affect running ability (such as stride, rhythm, injuries and so on)? I never previously detected the imbalance when running. Do I need a heel lift and, if so, how high and should it be placed inside the shoe or on the outside?

A: Leg-length discrepancy is more frequently present than it is symptomatic. Unless it bothers you in some way, giving knee or hip pain (frequently on the opposite side), I would not bother treating it.

In treatment, I think the lift should be placed inside the shoe. Correction should never be more than a half-inch, and not the total of one inch you found.

Chapter 11
Shoes and Inserts

IF THE SHOE FITS...

The worst thing that ever happened to feet was shoes—or perhaps the second worst, after concrete. These two products of urban civilization have finally conquered the human foot which, in its primitive state, crossed continents, pursued wild game and danced for days on end.

You may not think of the foot as man's crowning glory, but it has been and is still capable of these incredible efforts. You may not think of the foot as reflecting the personality of the owner, but it remains a key to the person's lifestyle and state of health.

This is especially true of the athlete. His feet determine not only his physiological fitness but his instability as well. Unfortunately, the far-reaching effects of foot trouble on the rest of the body are not generally realized by the medical profession or even by the podiatrists who make diseases of the foot their specialty.

The foot bone, so the song goes, is connected to the ankle bone, and the ankle bone is connected to the leg bone, and the leg bone is connected to the thigh bone, and the thigh bone is connected to the hip bone, and the hip bone is connected to the back bone. So hear the word of the Lord! The foot bone is where we start to come apart.

The motto of sports physicians then should be, "Look to the athlete's feet regardless of his complaints."

There is Biblical evidence for such an approach. "The head cannot say to the feet, I have no need of thee!" says Paul in First Corinthians. "God has so adjusted the body that there may be no discord. If one member suffers, all suffer together; if one member is honored, all rejoice together."

Abraham Lincoln put it this way: "When my feet hurt, I can't think." Lincoln's blunt Anglo-Saxon makes more evident Paul's philosophic statement. It reaffirms the body-mind synthesis and emphasizes, if it needs any emphasis, that man is his body.

It also tells us a universal truth: Painful feet affect saint and sinner, president and ward heeler, plodder and Olympian. And it reveals, since it implies a repeated event, that the Great Emancipator did more or less what we all do when we have trouble with our feet—nothing.

This resignation to the inevitable, this surrender to the belief that bad, weak and aching feet are just more evidence of man's frailty has carried over to the present day. I think it was Joan Crawford who asked, "Why is it when you say your foot hurts, it sounds all right, but when you say your *feet* hurt, it sounds lousy?"

It sounds lousy because it contains the implication that your feet—and, therefore, all the rest of you—are made of bad material; that life, as you are living it, has proven you inadequate—and, furthermore, nothing can be done about it.

It is not true. The material is good. Shoes and concrete have done us in, that and transportation. "Civilized man," wrote Emerson, "has built a coach and lost the use of his feet."

Brian Mitchell, a British national track coach, said recently that he could go through his entire working day and walk less than 100 yards. Over the centuries, feet have always been able to adapt, but not to inactivity.

But Lincoln's aching feet were the feet of an athlete. At 22, he weighed 180 pounds and was able, it was said, to outrun, outlift and outwrestle any man in Sangamon County, Ill. He once walked 34 miles in one day just to hear a famous lawyer argue a case in court. So Abe was no weekend athlete with a few blisters to show for overactivity. He was a counterpart of our present-day athletes who are paying the cost of ignoring their feet.

"The feet are unquestionably the most abused and neglected part of the body," states Harvard trainer Jack Fadden. "They do the most work and receive the least attention. And the major reasons for foot problems, of course, are shoes." The greatest asset an athlete can have, according to Fadden, is a well-fitted pair of shoes.

THE BEST SHOES

Q: What is the best shoe to wear?

A: I think it would be instructive to find how many runners use odd types of footgear without any difficulties.

When I first started running about 25% of runners used Tiger Cortez (now called Corsair). Many of the rest used sneakers, Hush puppies, garage mechanic shoes and the like. I recall I shifted to the New Balance Huntington which looked like a crepe-soled leisure shoe and even had a regular heel.

As the shoes got "better," it seems that the injuries increased. The better the changes are for one type of disorder, the worse they are for another. There is always a trade-off. The shoe good for controlling a hypermobile, flattening foot may cause trouble for a high-arched, rigid foot.

Other features like the undercut heel mystify me. They just mean trouble for certain people and don't help performance in others.

I have seen instances where the runner had gone the route with exercises and podiatry—only to be saved by a change in shoes.

Such changes should be intelligent. Many models are almost identical from company to company. You have to shift to a radically different type of shoe. Often, you can modify your own by grinding off the flanges of the heel, cutting the forefoot to increase flexibility or adding more shock absorption.

WIDER HEELS

Q: Some of the new shoes featuring wider and wider heels suggest stability and, therefore, fewer injuries. But some runners I know have experienced knee, calf and tendon problems after shifting to a wider heel style. Could the wider heels be causing more torsion to the lower leg?

A: Your comments are in agreement with a general experience. Many runners are getting into trouble with these shoes. The reason is still not known. However, one cause may be *too much* stability. The foot has to move to absorb shock and may not be able to do so with a wide heel. You might try trimming off the flange so the shoes don't have to be discarded.

HEEL HEIGHT

Q: I have been using a flat-bottomed, no-heel-elevation running shoe for many years. Recently, I have had tenderness and swelling of the Achilles tendon sheath. I switched over to a pair of shoes with some heel elevation, and this seems to have done the trick. Now I'm curious: Does a slight heel elevation really make that much difference in Achilles tendon strain?

A: Your experience is not unique. Achilles tendinitis can occur with what appear to be insignificant changes in heel elevation. I am now running with a low-grade tendinitis because I'm too lazy to have the heel of my shoes repaired. The first of the three rubber layers has worn through, a matter of only a quarter-inch. I had similar Achilles problems after one Boston Marathon because I used racing flats instead of my higher-heeled training shoes.

RACING SHOES

Q: Out of habit, I will do pre- and post-race stretching exercises along with running. However, the morning after a race (and to a lesser degree, after intervals) I inevitably experience an extreme tightness in my lower calves and achilles, and a tenderness beneath the bottom edge of my heels. I train in good running shoes, and my racing flats feel super. Any suggestions to eliminate the post-race pain?

A: The obvious solution is to wear your training shoes for your interval work and races. Many runners now do. I see more and more training shoes, especially in marathons and the longer races. Racing flats are usually weak on shock absorption, support and control.

A final word: We peak in performance perhaps three or four times a year. Why not reserve your racing flats for those extremely few meets and stay healthy in between?

TENNIS SHOES

Q: An orthopedic specialist who is a friend of mine told me that you recommended a certain type of shoe for running. I have been doing two miles daily for some 20 years using my tennis shoes. Could you suggest a type of shoe?

A: Let well enough alone. If you've had no discomfort with your tennis shoes, don't risk a change. The best shoe is the one that gives you no trouble, and you've already found yours. Enjoy your running and your tennis shoes.

SHOE REPAIR

Q: The glue gun that many of us are now using to repair the worn-down sides and backs of our running shoes has meant an enormous saving in time and expense. Since I've been doing this repair work, however, I have had several occurrences of swelling above the ankles. Could this be caused by the rebuilding of the heel and perhaps adding too much of a "lift" to the heel?

A: Your experience confirms what I've been trying to say here for years: In the footstrike, millimeters count. Joe Henderson, author of the original article on shoe-glueing, suggests now that best results are obtained by using the smallest possible amount of glue and spreading it smooth and "paper-thin" with the hot glue gun nozzle.

NO SUPPORT

Q: I have a problem with shoes giving my feet too much support. At the end of a run, I usually would have sore arches and some Achilles pain. The arch supports built into the shoes, no matter how soft, would feel like small cement blocks after a run. I removed the arch supports and now run without discomfort. Would running without arch supports lead to any long term complications?

A: Supports are like any form of therapy. Anything you put into the shoe has the possibility of making you worse than better.

Usually, it is the hypermobile, pronating foot that needs control. Such feet, however, can be over-controlled or restricted. Then, symptoms occur, usually on the outside of the foot, leg, knee and hip.

The high-arched, rigid foot often rebels against any control at all. It needs some movement in order to handle shock impact. Your story suggests that you have that sort of foot.

ORTHOTICS

Q: Could you discuss the pros and cons of "Sporthotics" (a brand-name orthotic or custom support) known thus far? I have a slight forefoot problem which makes me a little more injury-prone than other runners. The total cost of going to a podiatrist and having a neutral foot cast made to be sent to the Sporthotics laboratory and to have the Sporthotics will, I understand, cost more than $100. Is it worth it? Has it improved people's running that much?

A: I think every runner should first be convinced that orthotics are worth the expense. The best way to do that is to first go the maximum route with exercises and over-the-counter arch supports.

If running is painful or impossible, the first thing to do is establish strength/flexibility imbalance.

Next, Dr. Scholl's Flexos, then Dr. Scholl's "610's" should be tried. If there is a shoulder drop, a quarter-inch felt heel lift in the opposite shoe may help.

If at this point you are still hurting, you should see a *sports* podiatrist or an orthopedic surgeon who has an interest in and makes his own molds. He may or may not use Sporthotics.

Flexible, non-compressible supports are the easiest to make, wear and modify. Rigids, the most difficult to make and wear, give the best control. However, for speed and lateral motion, they are inferior.

Sporthotics attempt to be both, and because of this take on the weaknesses of both. They also tend to compress through the arch.

Still, when you get on the road, the effectiveness of the support probably relates more to the skill and experience of the sports podiatrist or orthopedic surgeon than to the specific type of orthotic.

Q: I've been injured and gone the way of orthotics as a possible cure. I was quite happy about this step until I read that you condemn orthotics. Is that still your stand?

A: Read that previous answer again. It was in response to a runner who wanted to know if orthotics were worth the money.

I said, of course, they are if you have exhausted other measures that will take care of 50% of our injuries—exercises and over-the-counter supports.

ARCH SUPPORTS

Q: While listening to speakers at the clinic preceding the Boston Marathon, I was tantalized by the mention of the Dr. Scholl's Athletic "A" and "610" supports. Where can I find these jewels?

A: The Dr. Scholl's company has designated six of its shops across the country as full-stock service centers or mailing centers for the "610" and "Athletic A" supports. Those stores are in Chicago, Ill. (21 North Wabash Avenue); Boston, Mass. (21-23 Temple Place); New York City (399 Fifth Avenue); Torrance, Calif. (160-A Del Amo Fashion Square); Birmingham, Ala. (211 North 21st Street); and Spokane, Wash. (419 Riverside). Officials for that company noted, however, that most of their stores do carry the supports.

ORTHOTIC FAILURE

Q: I began having knee trouble on the large tendon below the patella several years ago. I went to a podiatrist and was cast for orthotics. The orthotics made the problem worse. Finally, I ran into an orthopedic surgeon who suspected adhesions (inflamed bits of tendon). He operated on me and removed the adhesions around the tendon sheath. Now, all the pain is gone, and I am running again. My doctor says this proves that orthotics are nothing but a fad. My questions to you are: Why did orthotics fail, and is my doctor correct in his opinions?

A: Orthotics fail for a number of reasons:

1. The "neutral position" of the foot (from which the orthotics are cast) is difficult to find and mold. When in doubt, the podiatrist should err by making too small a correction.

2. Some runners can't stand full correction because their flexibility is greatly impaired.

3. The rear-foot correction with the rigid (usually plastic) orthotics is sometimes excessive. This causes jarring.

4. All rigid orthotics need adjustment. Runners may have to make several follow-up visits to get complete satisfaction.

5. Rigids are satisfactory at training speeds, but soft orthotics are usually necessary for competition, field events and very rough footing.

So it seems a badly fitted orthotic can make you worse as well as better. If the foot had nothing to do with the knee—as many orthopedists feel—then nothing you could put in the shoe would affect it either way.

Chapter 12
Extra Exercises

Training overdevelops the prime-movers—those muscles along the back of the leg and thigh and low back become short and inflexible. The antagonists—the muscles on the front of the leg and thigh and abdomen—become relatively weak. The following exercises, the "Magic Six," correct this imbalance:

1. The first stretching exercise is the *wall pushup* for the calf muscles. Stand flat-footed about three feet from the wall. Lean in until it hurts, keeping the knees locked, the legs straight and the feet flat. Count "one elephant, two elephants," etc. Hold for 10 elephants. Relax. Repeat for one minute.

2. The second is the *hamstring stretch.* Put your straight leg with knee locked on a footstool, later a chair and finally a table as you improve. Keep the other leg straight with knee locked. Bring your head toward the knee of the extended leg until it hurts. Hold for 10 elephants. Relax. Repeat for one minute, then do the same exercise with the other leg.

3. The final stretching exercise is the *backover* for the hamstrings and low back. Lie on the floor. Bring straight legs over your head and try to touch the floor with your toes until it hurts. Hold for 10 elephants. Relax by bringing your knees to your ears for 10 elephants. Repeat stretch and relax periods for one minute.

4. The first strengthening exercise is for the *shin muscles.* Sit

on a table with the legs hanging down. Put a 3-5-pound weight over the toes. Flex foot at ankle. Hold for six elephants. Relax. Repeat for one minute with each leg.

5. The second is for the *quadriceps* (thigh muscles). Assume the same position with the weight. This time, straighten the leg, locking the knee. Hold for six elephants. Relax. Repeat for one minute, and then do the same with the other leg.

6. The final exercise is the *bent-leg situp.* Lie on the floor with your knees bent and your feet close to your buttocks. Come to a sitting position. Lie back. Repeat until you can't do any more or have reached 20.

THE MAGIC SIX
Drawings by Nora Sheehan

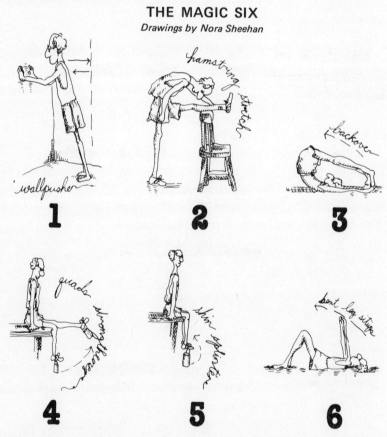

It takes a little over six minutes to do the Magic Six. Done before and after running, this means just 12 minutes a day to keep you in muscle balance.

VICTIM OF EXERCISE

Q: I am a "Magic Six" victim. I pulled my hamstring muscle doing the "backover." It took about six weeks to recover. It happened because I swung my leg over as if I were doing a gymnastic event. Now, I do yoga insteaad.

I don't recommend others shying away from the backover. What I do recommend is caution in doing it. Do it slowly. Haste can waste you.

A: All stretching should be done with the speed of a glacier and the patience of a yogi. You must approach the area of discomfort and then back off, then approach it again. No sudden movements should be made, nor should actual pain be experienced.

ACTIVE STRETCHES

Q: You advise against doing stretches in a bouncing manner. Instead, you advise stretching a muscle slowly until tightness sets in, holding for 10 seconds or so and then relaxing.

I have used the bounce method for some 20 or 25 years with satisfactory results. A few months ago, I decided to try your recommendation, but I soon went back to my old ways. The slow stretch method, I found, does stretch the muscle, but it does not loosen up the muscle in the sense of getting it to the point of contracting and relaxing swiftly and painlessly. By contrast, the bounce method both stretches and loosens. Since I am just as much interested in loosening as in stretching when I do my warmup exercises, I prefer bouncing.

Intuitively, it seems to be that slow stretching cannot be enough. In running, the muscles have to flex rapidly. Something has to be done to prepare for that, whether it be exercises or preliminary jogging. It also seems to me that if bouncing should be avoided, then people should never run. It is, after all, a bounce form of exercise.

A: I am a very poor stretcher myself. I rarely stretch unless I get into some painful condition with my back, calves or hamstrings. My advice, therefore, comes from some champion stretchers like Paul Uram, Ian Jackson, Bob Anderson and Karl Klein. I am also relaying the conventional wisdom found in most physiology texts.

I realize that what works for some people doesn't work for others. You have found bouncing works for you. However, if running is indeed a bouncing exercise, your theory is wrong. There can be no doubt that running tightens up the prime-movers. Try running twice a day without intervening stretching exercise.

MUSCLE BALANCING

Q: Lately, I have read of the need for balanced muscular development. Occasionally, I ride my bike to and from work. My question is, will riding a bike about four miles help or hinder running? I know it is not likely to hurt one's conditioning, but what about its effect on the muscles?

A: Bicycling is a fine way to maintain cardio-pulmonary conditioning—usually two miles of bike being equal to one mile of running. The muscles used in biking are different, however. The quadriceps get a good deal more action while riding, as do the muscles on the front of the leg.

Muscle balance can be established better with exercises for the anti-gravity muscles—shins, quads and stomach—done on a regular basis. Running backward is a trick. Some half-court basketball would be a more enjoyable way of doing it.

Q: After reading that running overbuilds certain muscles, I thought how ideal Emile Puttemans' job is for a runner. Puttemans (former world 5000-meter record-holder from Belgium) is a gardener who must bend over a lot in his work, which is the same sort of exercise one gets from doing bent-leg situps, Do you agree that gardening is beneficial in this way?

A: Yes. And I might add that gardening is also fine for the soul, adding something that bent-leg situps will never provide.

ARM TENSION

Q: I have noted that in the late stages of my races, I tighten up in my arms. Would you please give me some ways of solving my problem? What about lifting weights?

A: This tendency to tighten up is universal. When I run on the track, I usually station someone to yell "relax" as I go by. By the time I get back to him, my shoulders and arms are all tensed up.

"Relax" is the word. From your hips up, your body is simply for balance and breathing. Weight lifting, however, may be worthwhile to prevent fatigue of the respiratory muscles.

PUSHUP POWER

Q: Do you consider pushups a good complementary exercise for runners, and is there any correlation between my running rate and pushup capacity?

A: Pushups are for weightmen and have, to my eyes, no bearing at all for distance runners. If pushups correlate with anything, it would be with your speed in short dashes. They have little or nothing to do with aerobic fitness.

WEIGHT TRAINING

Q: I run on the track team at high school. I heard that ankle weights are not good to wear when you run. What is your opinion?

A: Ankle weights might cause an unnatural stride and, therefore, cause injury. However, there are advantages, both psychological and physical.

In college, I sometimes trained in high-top sneakers. When I wore spikes, I felt as if I had taken on wings. The physical advantage is that you may well be building up your own anti-gravity muscles, especially if you live where you can't do much hill work.

Q: I am a high school runner who is doing 15-20 miles a day. I want also to start lifting weights but am wondering if this will be too much of a strain on my body with the amount of running I'm already doing. Or will it help my running?

A: I have never been impressed with the value of weight lifting for distance runners. Proper form dictates that the body from the hips up is used for balance. There seems to be little need for strength.

I recall that Tom O'Hara (who once held the indoor mile record at 3:56.2) said he could only do three pushups. Since then, I have not concerned myself with weight training.

Nevertheless, I know of no reason these exercises should be harmful. They are not that demanding and can be done in association with a rigorous training program.

REBUILDING

Q: I am 10 weeks in a full leg cast. What is the best way to build up the thigh and calf muscles for a return to distance running?

A: I am going to give you an unorthodox answer to what appears to be a simple question.

The usual reply would be weight training. And, to an extent, that restoration of strength is necessary. However, a distance runner's leg muscles are predominantly slow-twitch endurance fibers, probably 75%. This means that a significant amount of rehabilitation must be one of the endurance type.

Therefore, I suggest you also use an exercise bike. This will aid in two ways. It will promote cardiopulmonary fitness and will retrain the endurance fibers of your legs.

Some laboratory work has been done by Dr. David Costill suggesting we may err in rehabilitation by making it almost all speed and strength exercises rather than combining them with endurance.

Chapter 13
Foot Injuries

WHAT GOES WRONG?

Overuse syndromes of the foot can be divided into these groups:

1. *Forefoot problems* include stress fractures (usually of the second or third metatarsal bones), Morton's syndrome (which differs from Morton's foot and is a term designated by neuroma of the metatarsal nerves, most commonly the third or fourth) and hallux rigidus (a painful condition of the big toe). Black toenails due to hemorrhages under the toenail are another problem of the forefoot, as are instances of metatarsalgia, sometimes called "bone bruises."

Forefoot injuries can occur in either the Morton's or high-arched foot, although stress fractures almost invariable occur in Morton's foot. Morton's neuroma occasionally responds to the usual measures involving shoes, surface, exercises, and store-bought or prescribed orthotics. However, it is one of the few instances where surgery may be the quickest and best treatment.

2. The main *midfoot injury* is plantar fascitis (which is most frequently associated with heel spur pain). Cuboid dislocations are rarely seen. But neuralgia can occur, as well as pain in the accessory scaphoid bone just below and forward of the ankle on the inside. Treatment must be directed to the use of supports, exercises and appropriate shoes.

3. The primary *rearfoot difficulty* is the heel spur syndrome (see Chapter 14), although nerve entrapments around the heel are also seen. It is important to remember here, as in most problems involving the foot, the specific area involved is usually the innocent victim of a totally failing foot. The heel spur is just the tip of the iceberg. The pull on the plantar fascia, itself stretched by a pronating arch, causes the pain. Hence, treatment has to be directed to the entire foot.

Each pain is characteristic. Stress fracture pain is often on the top of the foot, almost the only cause of severe pain on the top of the foot. X-rays are frequently negative and take as long as six weeks to show the callus that gives the diagnosis away. If necessary, a bone scan can be done to show the fracture.

Neuroma pain comes and goes. It is typically between the bones, and runs up to one or more toes. Bone bruises are usually metatarsal pain and can be relieved by a metatarsal pad or strapping.

TOE LENGTHS

Q: I have had eight months of pain in the ball of my foot, just back of the second toe. My second toe is longer than the big toe. My podiatrist says I have an interdigital neuroma and may need surgery.

A: People with your type of foot have a short first metatarsal bone, and the second metatarsal accepts much more than its share of the body weight. I think this is sufficient to account for your symptoms. There is no need to add the presence of a nerve tumor to explain the pain.

A study of foot loads (J. R. Scott, et al., *Journal of Bone and Joint Surgery*, May 1973) mentioned that at one point in running the first metatarsal head took almost 100% of the body weight. The second metatarsal head ordinarily bears up to 40% at one point. However, when the second is lengthened, those figures are probably reversed. This can cause pain, stress fractures, arch strains or foot pronation with all their attendant consequences.

I would advise an orthotic fashioned to distribute the weight better. It should have a Morton's extension and some arrangement to bear weight behind the second metatarsal head.

RIGID TOE

Q: Last year, I began having problems with my left big toe. The pain became so intense that I laid off for eight months. When I started again, the pain was still present. A podiatrist and a bone specialist both have diagnosed hallus rigidus, which means degenerative arthritis and calcium deposits in the big toe.

One doctor recommends removal of the calcium deposits, and the other wants to replace my defective joint with an artificial one. I want to run for the rest of my life. Will this surgery help me accomplish that goal?

A: Hallux rigidus usually can be handled by simply putting a rocker sole in your shoe. This is a regular neoprene sole about a quarter-inch thick which is applied to the entire shoe. Then, beginning at the ball of the foot, it is tapered to zero. This treatment is simple and can be effective in a number of problems with the forefoot or toes.

As usual, there are a number of surgical procedures to correct hallux rigidus. There is a surgical cure for almost everything. However, I feel all other avenues should be exhausted (as quickly as possible, of course) before surgery is accepted.

MISSING TOE

Q: I am a 56-year-old who was running 10 miles every other day until recently. Then, I had a run-in with my lawn mower and lost the big toe on my left foot. Now, I am wondering how that loss may affect my running. Just how important is a big toe to a runner? Will it make the pounding on the next toe worse or what?

A: My sports podiatry colleague, Dr. Richard Schuster, tells me he sees about one such injury a week. He assures me that nothing needs to be done. If you develop a callus in the area just behind the missing toe, a podiatrist can make a rocker sole for you. This is an extra quarter-inch sole with the area cut out where the callus is forming.

ARTHRITIC TOE

Q: I had been an active runner for about four years when I started having problems with my foot at the main joint with the big toe. This problem occurred after an intensive training period in which I had progressed to a 4:07 mile.

Now, the pain is more severe and is with me all the time, but becomes more pronounced after running. For that reason, I have been running very infrequently and substituting bicycling and other forms of exercise.

My problem has been diagnosed as degenerative arthritis plus bone spurs, and I have been told that surgery is the only corrective action possible. Is this toe joint problem common with runners? It is not, apparently, a well-publicized complaint.

A: Difficulty with the first metatarsal phalangeal joint is not uncommon in runners. It is also the joint most commonly involved in acute gouty arthritis.

The treatment is corrective supports (orthotics) for your foot. Usually, there is a failing foot and the big toe joint is only one of the structures in the foot affected. This could be a simple commercial arch support or a personally-molded support made by a sports podiatrist.

BUNIONS

Q: For the past four months, I have had pain on the inner border of my foot at the beginning of my big toe. The doctor says I have a bunion which should be removed. It is quite swollen and getting no better. What should I do? I have had to stop running and playing tennis because of the pain. Is surgery the answer?

A: Surgery is rarely the answer in foot disorders. The surgical procedure is usually cosmetic. It improves the appearance of the foot but does not get to the real cause. A bunion indicates abnormal foot function. It is, therefore, the result, not the cause, of the difficulty. Removing it is useless because the basic problem in the foot, faulty biomechanics, will not be corrected by the operation.

What you need is a functional evaluation of the foot. Most likely you have Morton's foot or its equivalent with a loose inner border. These cause abnormal weight bearing.

FLAT FEET

Q: While coaching cross-country this year, I've worked with a runner who has flat feet. His feet have no arches at all. In spite of this, he runs well. He seldom complains of pain or discomfort. Is there positive action we can take to prevent future trouble?

A: I see nothing to be gained by anticipating trouble that may never occur. For reasons obscure to me, many people have extremely flat feet yet have no symptoms. I would recommend no treatment except for the use of a good training shoe. As the runner gets heavier and into more distance, his feet may become symptomatic. At that point, a heel stabilizer and perhaps a longitudinal arch support might help.

ARCHES

Q: About two months ago, my longitudinal arch fell and I pulled a tendon in my ankle. I have had custom arch supports made, I have frozen my ankle three times a day, I have taped my arches, my ankles and just about everything else I could reach, and I have rested for 10-, 15- and 20-day periods. Yet nothing seems to help. What can I do about it? Lord, I'm going absolutely insane with inactivity!

A: From the amount of pain and discomfort you have, it appears that your plantar fascia is in bad trouble. This is usually the last stage in a foot that has been threatening to be in trouble for a long time.

I am surprised, however, that your custom arch supports did not help. I would not give up on podiatric help. Nothing else is going to get to your root problem, which is a biomechanically weak foot.

Q: I developed a sore right arch, so I bought a new pair of running shoes and added an arch support. My arch got better, but it is still sore. Should I continue to run on it, or should I give it a rest?

A: Arch supports are like eye glasses. Some people can walk into Woolworth's and buy a pair of glasses for less than $5 and be well fitted. Others have to get individualized lenses at considerable expense. The same situation occurs with arch supports.

If your arches don't work well, consult a sportswise podiatrist.

STRESS FRACTURE

Q: Recently, I ran in a marathon and at about the 13-mile point developed an incredible feeling of tightness in both calf muscles. I managed to complete the marathon after slowing down. However, the tightness persisted after the marathon.

Several days after the marathon, the outer edge of the ball of my foot became extremely sore. It has been almost a month since the marathon, and the foot soreness has still kept me from running. How can I alleviate the soreness, and what caused it?

A: My bet is that you have a stress fracture of the foot. The severe cramp you developed was your body's attempt to prevent further injury. Oddly, at that time you felt no pain in your foot.

Such a reaction is not unheard of. One woman runner told me she was running with a limp but no pain for some months before her physician picked up a stress fracture of the hip bone.

Such injuries do, of course, presuppose some precipitating biomechanical problem, either a weak foot or a strength/flexibility imbalance of the muscles, or both.

Chapter 14
Heel Injuries

HEEL SPUR

Q: What is a heel spur?

A: A heel spur is an extrusion of bone on the under surface of the heel. It is also thought, incorrectly, to be the cause of heel pain which is worse during and immediately after activity, and on arising in the morning. The pain feels like a nail sticking into the foot or a feeling frequently described as "stone bruise."

Q: If the heel spur doesn't cause this pain, what does?

A: Strain of the plantar fascia and inflammation at its insertion to the heel. The plantar fascia is the bowstring of the arch of the foot. It is a dense sheet of tissue that extends, fan-shaped, from the toes, narrowing down to anchor at the heel. The heel spur, therefore, is the innocent victim of a strained plantar fascia.

Q: What causes strain on the plantar fascia?

A: Any combination of events that causes the arch to flatten or pronate will put excessive strain on the plantar fascia. In common with most overuse syndromes of the foot, leg and knee, this means structurally weak feet, strength/flexibility imbalance, inadequate shoes, hard surfaces and excessive time or intensity of training.

Q: The heel spur syndrome, then, is an indication that the entire foot is failing?

A: Exactly. Given a weak foot, tight inflexible calf muscles, the 5000 footstrikes an hour you get in running games, poor shoes and an unyielding running surface, the foot begins to function abnormally and finally fails. If the fascia is strong, the abnormal forces may result in Achilles tendinitis or runner's knee or some other problem. But when the fascia fails to carry the load, heel pain occurs.

Q: What do you mean by a weak foot?

A: A weak foot is structurally inadequate to its task of balancing the forefoot and the rearfoot, and distributing weight on the forefoot. The most common weak foot is the Morton's foot. The inner border of this foot is lax. In footstrike and weight-bearing, it takes up the burden late, thereby imposing a major part of the work inappropriately on the other metatarsal bones. The result is collapse, pronation, flattening—whatever you want to call it. An abnormal torsion or twist is set up ascending through the foot to the leg, knee, hip and beyond.

Q: How does muscle tightness contribute to the heel spur pain?

A: The runner at full footplant comes forward about 10 degrees past the perpendicular over his foot. If the muscle can't give him this 10 degrees (and in 95% of runners, it can't), that movement comes through further flattening or collapsing of his arch. Training which increases this tightness and further shortens the prime-movers, therefore, increases rather than decreases the susceptibility to heel spur problems.

Q: How should I treat my plantar fascitis or heel spur syndrome?

A: Since your problem is a totally failing foot, the treatment must be total and directed to each aspect already mentioned.

Start with a good shoe. This should have a good heel counter, a relatively high heel, solid shank and a multi-layered sole.

Use a Dr. Scholl's "610" arch support. This can only be

obtained from a Dr. Scholl's shoe store or the home office in Chicago.

Add a quarter- to a half-inch surgical felt or sponge rubber heel lift hollowed out like a doughnut to take pressure off the tender area.

Do wall pushups and backovers to stretch your calves and hamstrings.

Run on grass and soft surfaces. Avoid speed and hill work.

Apply heat to the heel before running and ice afterward.

Q: My physician has suggested butazolidine and cortisone shots. What do you think about them?

A: Such drug treatments are only temporary pain-relievers. They treat the effects, not the cause. As soon as activity is resumed, the pain will come back. Pain-free running requires restoration of the architectural balance of the foot and leg through the use of supports and exercise.

Q: If I take all the steps you recommend and still have pain, what then?

A: See a competent sports podiatrist who has treated a number of athletes. He will be able to review your shoes, training and muscle status, and diagnose your foot problem. Then, he can give you tailor-made supports designed for your feet. Every foot is different, and the Scholl's support is often not fully effective.

SPUR SURGERY

Q: Would you comment on a recent Associated Press article which describes a new method of surgery for heel spurs?

A: Dr. Richard Schuster, who has now taken care of more than 1000 runners, tells me he has yet to treat a heel spur problem that didn't respond to properly made orthotics and appropriate exercises. He has yet to see a patient who has required surgery. (It is, of course, entirely possible that some people went elsewhere for help and did eventually have surgery.)

Heel spur problems require complete biomechanical evaluation of the foot, and prescription of corrective appliances. The heel is the innocent victim. Treating it is treating the effect, not the cause. This type of surgery may work, but only for spectators—not for athletes.

HEEL BRUISE

Q: A few months ago, I bruised my heels while running on a cinder track. I think the reason for this is that I was wearing shoes without enough padding in the heels. I stopped running for three weeks, and the soreness went away. But just recently I bruised my heels again. What could be causing this, and what can I do for it?

A: Good racing shoes are poor *training* shoes. They have poor shock absorption. If you have a weak foot, they will let you know it. I suspect you have such a weakness in your foot which is causing a strain on the arch. The pain occurs where the bowstring of the arch is attached at the heel. Most runners have tight Achilles tendons and hamstring muscles which make the strain on the arch even worse.

I suggest you do the following: (1) start flexibility exercises for your Achilles and hamstrings; (2) get a pair of well-supported shoes to train in; (3) get a pair of Dr. Scholl's "Athletic A" supports to put in the shoes; (4) cover the arch and the rest of the sole with quarter-inch surgical felt; (5) cut a hole in the felt where the heel is tender; and (6) transfer this pad from your running shoes to your regular shoes so you use it all the time.

Chapter 15
Achilles Injuries

TENDINITIS

Q: What is Achilles tendinitis?

A: It is an inflammation of the heel cord and/or the sheath that covers it. The tendon is tender to touch and usually thicker than the normal one. Running and even walking are painful.

Q: How often does Achilles tendinitis occur?

A: This is a disease of athletes, mainly those in the running sports. In a poll of 1000 runners by *Runner's World*, 12% reported disabling attacks of heel cord pain lasting two weeks or longer. It is also fairly common in tennis players, soccer players, handball players and to a lesser extent in basketball players.

Q: What causes this problem?

A: Achilles tendinitis has two fundamental causes—one muscular, the other structural.

The muscular cause is short, inflexible calf muscles which develop from prolonged participation in the athlete's sport. The tendon then attempts to compensate for this limited range. Any sudden stress or strain from footstrike to takeoff must also be absorbed by the heel cord itself. Unfortunately, about 90% of runners have abnormally short, inflexible calf muscles.

The structural cause of Achilles tendinitis is weak feet. The most common is Morton's foot. Other indicators of weak feet would be a history of having to wear corrective shoes as a child, or having "weak ankles," or Hagland's deformity (a bump on either side of the back of the heel). This is a sign of an unstable heel and the presence of an abnormal strain on the heel cord.

Q: What usually precipitates an attack of Achilles tendinitis?

A: Increased training, speed work, hill work, allowing shoes to run down at the heels, or a change of shoes can put excessive stress on the short calf and weak foot. Acute symptoms will then occur.

I once ran in a five-mile race in indoor running shoes with no heels. I thought I would never run again, the pain and swelling of the tendons were so bad.

I have also developed pain and tenderness during training from letting my heels wear down just a quarter of an inch.

Racing, since it introduces several of these factors (light shoes with little support and low heels, plus speed and hills and intense effort), is often followed by some amount of achilles difficulty.

Q: Can Achilles tendinitis be prevented?

A: Yes. First, you must correct the short calf muscles. This can be done by daily stretching both before and after running. You should also wear a shoe with an adequate heel elevation to compensate for the tight muscles.

Second, you must correct any instability in the foot. This may be done with a Dr. Scholl's "610" support (available at a Scholl's shoe outlet) or the use of a flexible, non-compressible support made from a mold by your podiatrist.

Q: Suppose I get Achilles tendinitis, what should I do?

A: Immediately, you should add a heel lift sufficient to make walking and then running pain-free. This may mean an inch or more of surgical felt.

Avoid hill and speed activity.

You should also run on the opposite side of the road or in the opposite direction on the track.

Try to run slightly pigeon-toed. This tends to tighten up the footstrike and minimizes strain on the heel cord. Ice the area after every workout.

At the same time, institute other preventive measures outlined above: exercises, shoes, etc.

Q: Will I be helped by medications, cortisone shots or whirl-pool treatments?

A: These are not remedies. They do not lengthen your calf muscles or correct your foot weakness or raise the heel on your shoes. As soon as you resume running, the pain will return. You have a problem in structural engineering. Drugs are, therefore, just a digression. In addition, cortisone shots may be followed by rupture of the tendon.

Q: I have gotten tailor-made supports, added heel lifts, done my exercises, worn the right shoes, and four months later I am still in trouble. What should I do?

A: You may be one of the tiny minority needing surgery. The sheath may be the problem, not the tendon. Opening of the tendon sheath and cutting of adhesions may help. Removal of a bony beak cutting into the tendon may also be needed.

However, surgery will be unsuccessful unless all the previously recommended measures are taken in the post-operative period. And it is quite possible that all you needed originally was more stretching, a higher heel and better foot control.

MY ACHILLES PROGRAM

Q: While recently increasing my weekly mileage in training for a marathon, I began having pain along my Achilles tendon. What can I do to cure this problem?

A: Achilles tendinitis frequently occurs after intensifying training, particularly with hill and speedwork. I seem to get my Achilles problems just before Boston Marathon races when I start into those kinds of workouts.

Once begun, Achilles tendinitis is the devil to get rid of. Going back to everything you were doing before—shoes, mileage, terrain, pace, etc.—doesn't seem to work.

My immediate reaction is to put enough heel lift in my shoes (I wear my Tiger Corsairs all day, every day) to make walking comfortable. Sometimes, this requires enough surgical felt to raise my ankle out of the shoe.

Next, I go to serious, easy, painless stretching. My usual daily stretching consists of bending over to tie my shoes. It has to be considerably more.

After the workout, I ice the area and in the evening I use contrast baths: first, as hot as I can stand it for 30-60 seconds, then as cold as I can stand it for a similar period. I keep this up for 15-20 minutes. You can use a hot tub if you wish and then use the plastic bag filled with crushed ice.

I also give up my shoes long enough to have the shoemaker put a new heel on. If I let that Corsair heel wear down to the second level, I begin to feel it in my Achilles.

If I think of it, I take a couple of aspirin before I run, to reduce inflammation.

Finally, as Mark Twain said, the tendinitis gets discouraged by all this activity and goes away.

ACHILLES SURGERY

Surgical treatment of Achilles tendosynovitis is advised by Dr. George Snook of the University of Massachusetts. Because of the failure of conservative therapy, he operated on three patients with satisfactory results.

During the operation, dense fibrous adhesions were found between the heel cord and the tendon sheath. These were divided by sharp dissection. The tendon sheath was not closed.

Running was resumed within 2½ weeks. No recurrence was noted in two years.

Dr. Snook's operation, plus new success with heel and arch supports, gives hope that chronic Achilles problems are on the way out. At present, a primary step is expert podiatric advice. If this is unavailing, surgical intervention of this sort seems relatively simple yet effective. Post-operative attention to basic foot problems is still necessary to prevent recurrence.

Chapter 16
Shin Injuries

SHIN SPLINTS

Q: What are shin splints?

A: Shin splints are pains in the anterior compartment of the lower leg. This is the area in the front of the leg between the two bones, the tibia and the fibula. The pain is worsened by rising on the toes or gripping the ground with the toes. The pain can range from mild to incapacitating. Fifteen percent of distance runners polled by *Runner's World* have had to lay off running completely at one time or another because of shin splints.

Q: When do shin splints usually occur?

A: The classic setting for shin splints is an unconditioned athlete early in the season of a sport demanding vigorous running or jumping on a hard surface. Where stop-and-go and change of direction are required, the possibility of shin splints increases. However, shin splints can also occur in well-conditioned endurance athletes such as distance runners when they switch to lighter shoes, hard surfaces, and speed or sprinting.

Q: What muscles and/or tendons are involved in shin splints?

A: The three muscles and tendons in the anterior compartment. One, the anterior tibial, lifts the foot and keeps it from flattening. The other two go with the toes. Together, they function in shock absorption and stabilization of the foot. Electrical studies have shown that they are the dominant muscles at the moment of pushoff. They are, therefore, intimately involved with acceleration.

Q: What is the basic cause of shin splints?

A: Overuse of these anterior compartment muscles. But as with all overuse syndromes, the demands of the sport are simply the precipitating element. The athlete's injury results from three basic factors: genes, training and environment. To understand this is to know how to treat shin splints.

Q: What is the genetic factor in shin splints?

A: A weak foot. Usually this is the Morton's foot. When the foot is weak or unstable, the anterior compartment muscles have to do more work.

Q: What is the training factor in shin splints?

A: The primary difficulty is that the anterior compartment muscles are relatively unused in ordinary running and endurance activity, and therefore become weak. Their opposing muscles, the calf muscles, become strong and tight and develop "dynamic contracture." This creates a strength/flexibility imbalance between prime-movers (gastrocs) and antagonists (anterior compartment muscles).

Q: What is the environmental factor in shin splints?

A: Shoes with low heels, poor shock absorption and no foot control are the major problems in this area. Hard surfaces are an additional hazard. Tennis players, for instance, are aware of the difference in symptoms going from asphalt to synthetic to grass courts.

Q: What is the immediate treatment of shin splints?

A: The proper treatment is ~~ice, elevation and rest.~~ The anterior compartment muscles are encased in a sheath like a sausage. Heat expands the injured muscles in an unyielding container and, therefore, increases the pain.

Q: What must the athlete do next to return to pain-free activity?

A: Correct the muscle imbalance. The primary problem here is to strengthen the anterior compartment muscles. The basic exercise is to sit on a table with the legs hanging over the sides and flex the foot to lift a weight (using a paint can or any weight system). At the same time, flexibility exercises of the calf muscle should be done. The best of these are wall pushups with the feet flat about three feet from the wall.

Q: What about the genetic factor, the weak foot?

A: Support and control of the weak foot may be needed, especially when exercise therapy is not curative. The heel must be stabilized, the arch supported and a crest put under the toes to keep them from gripping the ground. A Dr. Scholl's "610" or "Athletic A" support may be sufficient.

Q: What changes should be made in the athlete's environment?

A: Shoes and surfaces are the problem here. If possible, the athlete should train on grass, and avoid hills and speedwork. A good training shoe with a firm heel counter, good heel seat, solid shank and multi-layered sole is recommended. A supplementary heel lift may be necessary until the calf muscle loosens.

TIBIAL TENDINITIS

Q: I am often bothered by a condition very similar to shin splints but on the insides of the calves rather than the fronts of the legs. I would appreciate information on this.

A: Your difficulty is with the posterior tibial muscle, its tendon and its attachment to the tibia. The tendon of this muscle goes under the inside ankle bone and then across under the arch to the base of the big toe. It thus forms a sling for the arch. When the foot pronates (flattens), it puts a strain on this tendon and pulls on the muscle, causing pain.

The solution is foot control—a support to stabilize the heel and keep the foot from pronating. I suggest you get a Dr. Scholl's "610" or "Athletic A" support to use all the time, running or not.

POSTURE

Q: Dr. Richard Schuster's opinion is that running more erect will help turn off shin splints. Would you suggest ways I may be able to change from a too-forward stance when I run?

A: The upright posture is the badge of Bill Bowerman's runners at the University of Oregon. It is a simple matter to switch to that running form. You "run from the hips" and use the upper body for balance. An additional help is to run with your toes "floating." Grabbing the ground with the toes seems to make shin splints worse.

SHIN SURGERY

Q: After I suffered from debilitating shin splints, I underwent surgery performed by Dr. George Snook of the Cooley-Dickinson Hospital, Northampton, Mass. He found adhesions between the tendon and tendon sheath above my right ankle. In both legs, he also released the fascia which was abnormally tight and thick, thus causing a painful condition.

Recovery was very swift (running within two weeks). It has been more than two years since the last operation (there were three), and I have not had a hint of shin pain since.

You have mentioned (Chapter 15) Dr. Snook's tendon operation for the Achilles. He has performed the fascia operation on several athletes. I hope other runners who suffer from these same injuries may soon benefit from surgery as I have.

A: Although I consider surgery as a last resort, if it had to be done, I would gladly consult Dr. Snook. In your case, you apparently had the end stage of those shin splints that have considerable tendinitis. In such instances, a grating is audible with a stethoscope and is even palpable when the foot is moved.

The use of corrective supports, Achilles stretching, etc., should prevent a runner with shin splint from reaching the "grade IV" condition you had. Still, it is good to have such surgical methods available when podiatric care and physiotherapy fail.

Chapter 17
Knee Injuries

MERRICK'S KNEES

Distance runner Dave Merrick's painful knees and how they were cured should be the sports medicine story of the decade. Not for the football people perhaps or the physicians whose weekly job it is to patch up those warriors for another game, but certainly for most of America's athletes young and old, daily and weekend, whose difficulties come from overuse, not from contact.

Merrick's knees are our knees. And what helped him will help us. Here is the story:

Merrick, a junior at the University of Pennsylvania and a 4:07 miler in high school, was being advised to have a second operation for the difficulties with his knees. He had been unable to train seriously for almost 14 months because of recurrent knee pains. During that time, the medical establishment in Philadelphia had taken its best shot to restore him to health. First rest, then exercises, then whirlpool, then drugs. Next, cortisone shots. Finally, a delicate operation in which the back of the kneecap was shaved. In every instance, as soon as he resumed training, the pain returned.

When surgery was offered the second time, Merrick and his coach Jim Tuppeny blew the whistle. Orthodoxy had been tried and found wanting. It was time to see a doctor who was a runner and might know something not in the books. They came to me.

They were not immediately impressed. "I thought Dr. Sheehan was nuts at first," Merrick told reporters. "I thought he was some kind of quack. Here, my knees are all swollen, and he's looking at my feet."

What I saw were two almost flat feet. No one had bothered to look at his feet on previous examinations or to ask about them. I did.

"I always wore corrective shoes when I was little," he said. "But then I started wearing loafers and got away from them."

So Merrick had weak feet and had always had them. Each time his foot hit the ground it flattened out and sent a short, quick twist up to the knee. This, in turn, pulled the kneecap out of its groove and irritated the cartilage. All he needed was someone to treat his feet. The knee would take care of itself.

In common with most doctors, I know little about the foot and even less about the foot in action. So I sent him to Dr. Richard Schuster, a podiatrist or specialist of the foot, who knows about the foot in action because he has treated more than 1000 athletes in the New York area.

This is most important. Even if you see feet day in and day out, examine them, diagnose them and prescribe for them, the athlete can be a difficult patient. He needs meticulous measurements, special care and frequent adjustments.

Schuster, whose patients include ballet dancers, cyclists and tennis players, gave Merrick that kind of examination and treatment. He made custom-fitted supports (orthotics). These maintained Dave's feet in the neutral position through footstrike and pushoff.

It was as if he had given Merrick wings. Within six weeks, he was in top form. He really began to roll during cross-country season, breaking course and meet records on four separate occasions. In November, he became the first man in history to break 24 minutes on the five-mile course at Van Cortlandt Park.

Merrick had passed the final test—prolonged pain-free running. As long as he wears his orthotics, he is "cured."

Merrick's 14 months of pain using traditional methods should not go unnoticed. We doctors keep using treatments that fail because we have nothing better to substitute for them. Now, that is no longer necessary in "runner's knee." There is a cure: treating the foot. And there is a man who can do this: the sports podiatrist.

RUNNER'S KNEE

Q: What is "runner's knee"?

A: Runner's knee (also known as tennis knee, jumper's knee, volleyballer's knee, etc.) is an erosion of the cartilage covering the underside of the kneecap. Chondromalacia of the patella, as it is known medically, causes pain in and around the front of the knee. It occurs during running, or going up and down stairs, after sitting for a while and then walking around.

Q: How frequent is runner's knee?

A: It is the most frequent overuse injury in all of sports and the most frequent complaint of runners. A *Runner's World* poll showed that 23% of runners had been sidelined for long periods of time with this problem. Sports podiatrist Dr. Richard Schuster reports that nearly 75% of runners seeking help have knee pain, although not always as the primary complaint.

Q: What is the cause of runner's knee?

A: Four factors occur singly or in combination to cause runner's knee:

1. Structural instability of the foot. Any tendency for the foot to pronate or flatten will produce this. Morton's foot is the most frequent foot abnormality found in association with runner's knee.

2. Postural instability. Short calf and hamstring muscles put further stress on the weak foot.

3. Leg-length discrepancy.

4. Environmental stresses. These include inadequate shoes and running on slanted surfaces which further stress the weak foot.

Q: How do these factors cause runner's knee?

A: Runner's knee begins with the foot. The structurally unstable foot flattens and causes the lower leg bone to twist to the inside. This "torsion," transmitted to the knee causes the kneecap to pull off center in the patellar groove of the thigh bone and consequently to ride over on the knob or condyle. This is repeated about 5000 times in an hour of running, and the resulting irritation produces pain.

The tight calf muscle increases the tendency of the arch to flatten, as does a shoe without support or shank. Running on the left hand side of the road will flatten the right arch, and the opposite effect occurs while running with traffic.

Q: What can be done for runner's knee?

A: You must treat the foot, not the knee. Treatment directed at the knee is a waste of time. Therefore, it is essential that treatment be directed at the four elements causing the difficulty:

1. Foot supports. These may be simple like Dr. Scholl's Flexos or may have to be individualized. The runner may have to see a podiatrist.
2. Flexibility exercises for calf and hamstring muscles.
3. Lifts to equalize leg lengths.
4. Good training shoes with a solid shank and multi-layered soles.

Q: What about cortisone shots, butazolidine, casts, rest, acupuncture or surgery for runner's knee?

A: All these treatments are symptomatic. They do not get to the cause of the disorder. If you want to return to pain-free running, you must treat the foot. Otherwise, you are treating the effect, not the cause.

Q: How soon should I feel relief with a foot support, exercises and proper shoes?

A: I have seen runners competing pain-free in 10 days. Usually, a few days will convince you that you are going in the right direction. If not, you may need further adjustment on the supports.

Q: Will this treatment also help tendinitis, Osgood-Schlatter's disease, torn cartilage or arthritis of the knee?

A: Whatever the disease of the knee, it will be helped by having the kneecap glide in its groove and keeping the knee functioning in its correct plane. Removing the torsion set up by an abnormal footstrike will frequently make pain-free running possible even in these conditions.

SELF-ANALYSIS

Q: About 2-3 miles into my daily run, the side of my right knee begins to get very painful. It seems I can postpone the pain by running slower and reducing my stride. Strangely, the pain almost immediately disappears after I stop running, with only a stiffness remaining. There is no swelling. Any help would be appreciated.

A: When any injury occurs, you should go though a systems analysis. Among the questions you might ask are:

1. *Have I changed shoes?*
2. *Have I let my old ones run down?*
3. *Have I increased my mileage?*
4. *Have I changed my terrain?*
5. *Have I changed my training routine?*
6. *Am I doing more speed work?*
7. *Did I race in racing shoes?*
8. *Am I running on a track?*
9. *Have I neglected my exercises?*

After that, you frequently can pinpoint the cause of your problem. Treatment usually involves shoe modification, exercises and over-the-counter arch supports.

Your injury incidentally, is runner's knee. Now start asking yourself those questions.

POST-RACE PAIN

Q: I developed chondromalacia of the knee last year, and as a result of using sport orthotics, the pain left completely. But three days after my last marathon, I developed the same problem, after months of trouble-free running. Can I develop the same problem again even with orthotics?

A: Injuries following marathons are quite common. Usually, the runner wears lighter shoes in the mistaken notion they will improve performance. What happens is they give neither support nor shock absorption.

The increase in training mileage for a marathon also causes problems, creating inflexibility and increasing foot stress.

TORN CARTILAGE

Q: I am a high school student who began running cross-country in the fall. I tore a cartilage in my right knee, possibly from overtraining. Should I have the cartilage removed?

A: I would not submit to cartilage surgery without an arthroscopy. This is a procedure where the doctor can actually look inside the knee and see what is going on.

In your instance, I would suspect you have a simple case of runner's knee, and may need nothing more than attention to your feet and diligence in doing stretching exercises.

KNEE SURGERY

Q: Recently, I had surgery on my right knee. Is there any way I can resume running as soon as possible but not at the cost of a knee?

A: My correspondence has made me quite optimistic about running after knee surgery. The pathology in the joint should be halted from progressing and even reversed if the knee joint is made to operate normally.

As you might suspect from reading what I've written, this means attention to the footstrike and any associated strength/flexibility imbalance of the muscles.

Q: I am slated for surgery for a torn cartilage in my knee. How long will it be before I get back to running?

A: A new technique for removal of torn cartilage fragments has been developed by Dr. David Dandy in England. It involves the use of the arthroscope and it is, according to Dandy, "difficult, tedious, often protracted and should be attempted by surgeons who have confidence in their arthroscopic techniques."

However, when done this way, return to work was reduced from a range of 38 to 90 days down to 10.5 days. Hospital stay averaged 1.3 days in Dandy's 30 patients.

Such surgery, however difficult, presents definite advantages for runners and other athletes, since time away from their sport will be minimized.

At present, since such surgery is available only on a limited basis, it appears as if a prolonged rehabilitation period will be necessary.

TENDINITIS

Q: For nearly six months, my knee has been aching. I don't think it's chondromalacia. My school trainer thinks it's tendinitis. I'd like to know the difference between the two and if tendinitis results from an imbalance of the foot.

Q: Most knee problems in runners are chondromalacia, even when they're called tendinitis. When tendinitis occurs, however, it develops for the same reason—a twist applied to the knee through each footstrike. As in chondromalacia, you must look to some imbalance in your foot, a shoe type with a weak shank that fails to support your midfoot, or excessive wear in the shoe.

LIGAMENT PAIN

Q: I have sharp pains in the ligaments on the outside of my knees. The pain seems to be relieved by stretching and lasts only a few days, so it's not crippling, but I would like to know what to do to stop the pain. I run 30-60 miles per week.

A: Outside knee pain is usually due to shock impact. This suggests a number of things: (1) a foot that does not handle shock well, the high-arched or cavus foot; (2) tight calf muscles which refuse to "give" and contribute to shock absorption; (3) shoes with not enough rubber up front or at the heel, i.e., those that test poorly for shock; (4) poor form where you are overextending by bringing your foot ahead of the neck; or (5) concrete or other hard surfaces that would accentuate any of the above problems.

You can see it will be necessary to take a total approach to this difficulty, including surface, shoes, exercises and running form.

OSGOOD-SCHLATTER'S

Q: I am a 19-year-old runner who has been averaging about 50 miles a week for the last four years. In the last six months, I have developed acorn-size knots on the bones of both my legs, approximately one inch below each knee. They cause me no pain or trouble most of the time, but are quite painful when I bang them against something hard. Occasionally, when I am out on a run of longer than five miles, they begin to ache and get sore, but not so bad that I have to stop. Should I be concerned?

A: You have Osgood-Schlatter's disease (an inflammation of the epiphysis, the growing center of the tibia in that area). When this epiphysis fuses to the bone, the pain will cease. In the meantime, continue to run within pain limits.

BAKER'S CYST

Q: My doctor tells me that I have a Baker's cyst on the back of my knee. I understand it is not caused by running, but running certainly aggravates the problem. Just what is a Baker's cyst, and what treatment do you suggest?

A: A Baker's cyst is an extension of the joint capsule of the knee. It is filled with joint fluid. Its appearance, therefore, means something is afoot with your knee.

Treatment of the Baker's cyst is to ignore it and treat the foot. Most knee problems arise from abnormal kinetic forces originating at footstrike, footplant or toeoff.

If this herniation or sac becomes quite painful, surgery might be considered. However, attention to biomechanics of the foot, plus muscle strength/flexibility imbalance should do the trick.

Chapter 18
Muscle Injuries

HAMSTRING PULLS

Steve Williams, the world's fastest human, and Marty Liquori, the country's best-known middle-distance runner, failed to make the 1976 Olympic team because of hamstring muscle pulls. This raised a number of questions about the injury.

Q: What is a hamstring pull?

A: A muscle pull is anything from a cramp to a disruption or a tear of the muscle-tendon-bone complex. It may occur in the belly of the muscle, or at its connection with its tendon, or at the tendon's attachment to the bone.

The hamstring is the muscle group that comprises the back of the thigh. The muscle that pulls, however, is usually the biceps femoris, a two-headed muscle which inserts on both the thigh bone and the pelvis.

Q: Why does a muscle pull?

A: A muscle pulls because it is too weak or too inflexible. A weak muscle pulls in the belly. A short, inflexible muscle pulls at its tendon or its connection with the bone. Any muscle will pull in its belly if maximally contracted and suddenly stretched.

Q: Do both types of pull occur in the hamstring?

A: Yes. The sprinter whose hamstrings are weaker than his quadriceps, the powerful front thigh muscles, pulls in the belly. We are familiar with the sight of a sprinter suddenly grasping the back of his thigh in the final stages of a 100-meter dash. The distance runner, on the other hand, has powerful, over-developed hamstrings he neglects to stretch. His pull consequently is in his buttocks where the long head of the biceps attaches to his ischial tuberosity.

Q: Has there been any scientific study to demonstrate that weakness of the hamstring versus the quadriceps causes hamstring pulls in athletes?

A: Lee Burkett at San Diego State tested 30 trackmen, 12 of whom had sustained hamstring pulls. The 12 all had one hamstring significantly weaker than the other. The other 18 had normal 60-40 quad hamstring strength ratios and no difference between the hamstrings.

He also tested 36 San Diego Charger football players and, on the basis of weak hamstrings, predicted that 6 would have pulls. Four did pull their hamstrings; a fifth developed early symptoms and was withdrawn from the study. None of the 30 rated as normal had pulls.

Burkett, therefore, concluded that the hamstring pulls could be predicted by a very simple testing technique used regularly during the season.

Q: If hamstring pulls can be predicted from either a change in the normal 60-40 quad/hamstring ratio or loss of flexibility, can anything be done to prevent them?

A: Of course. Paul Uram, formerly with the Washington Redskins and now "flex coach" of the Pittsburgh Steelers, has proven that a program of testing and remedial exercises virtually will eliminate the problem of hamstring pulls. In his two years with the 'Skins and first three years with the Steelers, only one player missed a game because of hamstring injury.

Q: What is Uram's program?

A: Each year the entire squad is tested and evaluated. Those whose quad/hamstring ratio is higher than 60-40 are placed on specific "resistive flexibility exercises." Uram regards a 70-30 ratio, for instance, as almost positive proof that the player will pull. Also, any history of previous injury puts the player in that special category that must do these exercises regularly. Uram, of course, has the entire Steeler squad doing his intensive flexibility program on a daily basis (the center can do a ballet split). The Steelers stretch before the game, at halftime and after the game. They also win Super Bowls.

Q: If hamstring pulls are predictable and preventable, why do they still occur?

A: Burkett and Uram have clearly demonstrated that hamstring pulls are not an act of God. They can be predicted by simple tests of quadriceps and hamstring strength and flexibility. They can be prevented by the daily use of a simple series of flexibility exercises. Their continuing and frequent occurrence in major league ball parks, as well as in college and high school sport, is due to the ignorance of those treating, training and coaching those athletes.

THIGH TIGHTNESS

Q: In a marathon, I picked up the pace at around 12 miles. My thighs tightened and by 20 miles were really hurting. It was a nice, cool day and at the end I really didn't feel very tired. At Boston, my thighs tightened up again. They started tightening at 5-6 miles and by 10 miles really hurt. There, I was trying to hold back on the early downhill part. I have run workouts that fast for 15 miles or better and my thighs didn't bother me.

A: Tightening of thighs can occur for a variety of reasons. One is, of course, the one you mentioned—checking your speed on a downhill course like Boston. Also in Boston that year, the heat would have been a definite factor in the tightness.

Shoes and surface can be problems, especially when you switch from shock-absorbing training shoes to racing shoes. In addition, running a marathon is nothing like a training run. The actual race seems to cause runners to tighten up, lose their form, and in general feel the distance and pace inappropriately.

I would recommend you study these factors: (1) fluid replacement; (2) shock absorption; (3) relaxation; (4) running form; (5) course topography.

I train on flat roads and find that after Boston or other hilly marathons I usually have to go downstairs backward for a few days because of quadriceps (front thigh) pain and tightness.

Q: I began running six years ago and have since done it on a daily basis. Now, I am in need of medical advice from a runner. Pain, numbness and a sensation of weight in my quadriceps has constricted my running. Efforts to relieve this problem—by halving my distance and eliminating intervals—do no good.

At one time, I suspected a potassium deficit, but blood tests showed my potassium level to be normal. The whole problem seems to be related to stress and overuse, yet I don't think my program has been too stressful.

A: I suspect that your daily mileage is too much for your body, legs, feet, shoes and surface to handle. Alteration of one or more of these could help.

You could eliminate hills or go into low gear if there is no other way around them. Do interval work and speed work only in preparation for three or four important races during the year. Make sure you have totally recovered from the previous day's workout (use basal pulse rate). Take at least one day off a week.

In addition, try to run on grass or dirt where possible, shorten your stride, and use good training shoes. Do your stretching exercises regularly.

You may not consider your program stressful, but your body does. The program caused you to break down. You must now make adjustments. If you return to the identical regimen, you will be certain to fall into the pit again.

CALF STRAIN

Q: I am a 36-year-old who has been running seriously for more than two years. I always have had what I felt to be good running shoes. My goal is to run a marathon, but whenever I go on training runs or races beyond 10 miles, I have rather marked strain in my gastrocnemius (calf) muscles.

This is almost always in the right leg. However, the left often appears somewhat strained as well. Twice in the past year, I have so severely pulled the right one that I had to stop running for two weeks and even had difficulty walking without marked pain.

Realizing the difficulty of diagnosis without examination, I still would like your expertise in this matter.

A: It may be the origin of your posterior tibial tendon that is giving you trouble. In any case, I think you need some stabilization of your heel and an arch support.

Inflexibility of your shoe sole may be contributing. Try cutting across the sole of the shoe with a razor at half-inch intervals, one in the shank, next in the junction with the ball of the shoe, then on the ball itself.

GROIN STRAIN

Q: I've been injured with a strained groin muscle for more than a month now and it's becoming frustrating. What stretching exercises, if any, can I do to help matters along?

A: Groin injuries are the worst. Usually, there is a problem in the foot plus poor shock absorption. The possibility of one leg being shorter than the other should also be considered. And there are almost always some weakness and tightness of the inside thigh muscle.

I suggest: good shock absorbing shoes, a quarter- to half-inch heel lift in the shoe on the good leg, and do the Magic Six exercises (see Chapter 12). An inside thigh muscle stretching exercise involves sitting with the soles of the feet opposing and pulling toward the groin.

MUSCLE CRAMPS

Q: It appears there are considerable cramps (or so-called "heat cramps") in long-distance runners, particularly during summer months. Factors such as muscle glycogen depletion, electrolyte depletion and lactic acid accumulation have been mentioned. What are your thoughts on this?

A: The cramps at the end of a marathon and the usual nocturnal cramp or charley horse are two different disorders and probably have different causes.

The marathon cramp is a generalized tightness and soreness of the legs. Once seated after a marathon, or on hands and knees as I have been on occasion, I have had to be pulled to the standing position. There is no knotting or localized spasm in the muscles. My own suspicion is that it is due to an accumulation of lactic acid or at any rate to some metabolites that I should have cleared out but are still there.

I had the other cramp or spasm only once, in a marathon. On that run, I drank a lot of tea and cola on a hot day. I blame it on a salt loss with the added caffeine.

Q: During two marathons in March, I suffered from severe leg cramps in the last four miles, and as a result my times were probably at least 10 minutes worse than they would have been otherwise. The following month, I ran at Boston and once again experienced leg muscle cramps after about 22 miles. This time, they were even more severe than before. I have run eight marathons in the last seven months. In the first five there were no signs of difficulty. What can be done to avoid these cramps?

A: Your difficulties are probably due to dehydration. My calculations put your fluid loss in the neighborhood of one gallon—the equivalent of nine pounds in weight. This is probably close to the dangerous level of 6% of your body weight, beyond which lurk heat exhaustion and heat stroke.

I suppose your difficulties in earlier marathons were also due to this dehydration, a dehydration possibly worsened by chronically low glycogen content in your muscles from overracing.

I recommend (1) supercompensation of glycogen with a high-starch diet 48 hours before your races, and (2) super-hydration with water and appropriate amounts of salt and potassium during the race. You will need at least a pint every 20 minutes to keep near your starting weight.

Adjust your fluid and electrolyte intake. Check your weight before and after these long races. Your problem should be resolved right there.

Q: About every 3-4 weeks, I'm awakened by a severe cramp in the calf muscle of one of my legs. I can't relate the cramps to the amount of running I've done that particular day. What causes the cramps, and what can be done to prevent them?

A: Night cramps have been a mystery to the medical profession over the centuries. Running by itself is not the cause. However, excessive daily mileage, dehydration, too much coffee, or a change in training to hill work and intervals may be precipitating factors.

The best prevention is probably regular flexibility exercises for the leg muscles. Vitamin E has been recommended, as has calcium supplementation. The best drug seems to be quinine. When used in five-grain doses at bedtime for a week or so, quinine will usually eliminate cramps for a long period. What may be happening, of course, is that the cramp has struck and left, to return 3-4 weeks later.

MUSCLE TWITCHES

Q: Two years ago, I developed fasciculations in both my legs, from below my knees to my toes, that have not ceased yet. A neurologist and two family internists just smile and shake their heads and say keep running. I wonder if any other runners have had similar problems.

A: Fasciculations, rippling of the muscles due to contractions, are a common finding in the hours following a long run. However, to my knowledge few runners have them continually. The exact cause of this muscle irritability is not known. Why you are even more susceptible is an even deeper mystery.

Fasciculations are no reason not to run. If more serious evidence of muscular irritation or even muscular destruction (dark brown urine) should occur, it would warrant investigation.

You might try good doses of vitamin C, calcium or vitamin E, all of which have been recommended for muscle cramps. It would be interesting to see if they have any effect.

Chapter 19
Back Injuries

SCIATICA

The sciatic nerve is the longest river of pain in the body. It arises from the nerve root of the fourth lumbar spine, an origin almost as obscure as the north end of Lake Itasca, the source of the mighty Mississippi.

But before long, this trickle is joined by the nerve root of the fifth lumbar spine, and then the roots of the first and second sacral spines. And now we have a nerve that can prevent sleep, destroy your personality and end a running career. It carries pain that varies from a discomfort to a catastrophe.

The medical books describe it as spontaneous, protracted, excruciating and intractable. If you have had sciatica, you know what that means, but you might substitute four-letter Anglo-Saxon words for the multisyllable Latin.

At least 10 million Americans live in Sciatica County, which stretches from Upper Buttocks to Foot Bottom. They live in little depressing towns called Agony and Woe, Ache and Throb, Torment and Torture. And like every inhabitant since Cotugno discovered sciatica in 1764, they are trying to escape. There is hardly a drug or device, operation or manipulation that hasn't been tried by these sufferers.

Now, their salvation may be at hand. Our athletes, who are otherwise normal—or even supernormal—individuals are getting sciatica. And in them at least, we can rule out these bizarre diseases in the textbooks and the onset of aging, which the

131

medical profession blames for everything that happens to us. Athletes are pointing the way to other explanations and solutions.

The athlete with sciatica may have low-back pain, but is more likely to have pain in the hip or in the leg from the hip to the big toe, or anywhere in between. At times, the sensation may be numbness, tingling or a feeling of "going to sleep" rather than pain. However, the cause of all these syndromes is the same. They result from a combination of:

• *Structural weakness:* Due to major or minor bony or ligamentous malalignments in the spine.

• *Postural weakness:* Due to overdevelopment of the back muscles and relative weakness of the stomach muscles.

If you know why you can do any number of situps with your legs flat on the floor but hardly any with your legs bent and feet on the floor, you'll know why you have low-back pain and sciatic nerve pain—and you'll know what to do about it.

Your overdeveloped, inflexible iliopsoas muscles make straight-leg situps easy. Your weak abdominals make bent leg situps impossible.

Because training increases the strength and tightness of the hamstrings and iliopsoas muscles while doing nothing for the stomach muscles, the experienced runner is more likely to develop these problems than the beginner.

Tightness of the achilles and gastrocnemius may also contribute to the backward rotation of the pubic bone, a characteristic finding in lordosis or "sway-back."

Speed work, in which the drive off the foot accentuates the arch of the back, is another frequent precipitating cause of sciatic difficulty.

The treatment is aimed at (1) flattening the spine; (2) rotating the pubic bone forward and the hips backward. Primarily, this is to be done by exercises to loosen up the iliopsoas, hamstring, and Achilles, and strengthen the abdominals. (Chapter 12 describes the recommended exercises, the Magic Six.)

Additional advice:

1. Go without shoes at home to stretch muscles in the back of the legs.

2. Sit with knees higher than hips.

3. Drive car with bucket seats.

4. Sleep on "good" side with knee of painful side drawn up toward chest.

5. Learn to live 24 hours a day without a hollow in the lower part of your back.

6. Use sacral support made by Futuro or Bellhorn (can be obtained at drugstore).

7. Check for discrepancy in leg length. Lifts for the short leg (and, oddly, at times for the long leg) may help.

8. Try osteopathic and chiropractic adjustments for *temporary* help.

9. Do not expect help from drugs, shots, whirlpool, acupuncture, etc.

LOW-BACK PAIN

Q: How important of a problem is low-back pain?

A: Impairment of the low back is the main cause of limitation of normal activity in the under-45 age group. "It is the condition," states Dr. Howard Rusk, "that causes more discomfort, more loss of time from work and disability than any other."

Q: What causes low-back pain?

A: As with sciatic nerve pain, this is a result of two factors. The first, structural instability, is due to congenital or acquired faults in the bones and ligaments. The second, postural instability, is due to strength/flexibility imbalance of the muscles.

Q: Where is the structural instability?

A: Most often at the lumbo-sacral junction. Often, x-rays disclose supposedly minor congenital abnormalities or the breakdown of the vertebral structure which usually occurs at or before the age of five years. In addition, two other forms of structural weakness are frequently encountered: (1) biomechanically weak feet, most often Morton's foot or some degree of flat feet, and (2) leg-length discrepancy, one leg shorter than the other.

Q: Where is the strength/flexibility imbalance?

A: Mostly between the spine and the belly muscles. Almost every low-back sufferer has weak stomach muscles. A study at Iowa University showed that the spine muscles of people with low-back pain were 9-10 times more powerful than their stomach muscles. In addition, athletes and especially runners overdevelop the iliopsoas, hamstrings and calf muscles. These become tight, short and inflexible, thus accentuating the sway back. Usually unrecognized is the fact that the tight calf muscle increases the tendency to flattening of the feet and, therefore, their bad effects on the spine.

Q: Can I test myself for this imbalance?

A: Quite easily. First try to do a bent-leg situp with your hands clasped behind your neck. That will settle your strength problem. For flexibility, there are three tests. To test the back muscles, stand with your back against the wall and flatten the hollow of your back. You should be barely able to get your hand in the space. (I have seen some people with room there for a fist.) To test the hamstrings, sit upright on a table with your legs extended, and see if it hurts the back of your legs. To test the calf, try to touch the floor without bending your knees.

Q: I have an abnormal x-ray, one leg is shorter than the other and I have a Morton's foot. What do I do?

A: The whole aim of treatment is to reposition the pelvis so the hips are back, the pubic bone forward, the back flattened. Your program might start with heelless or negative-heeled shoes. They shift the center of gravity back toward the hip joint. Next, wear a small, light back support. One such is the Futuro Sacrogard obtainable at the drugstore. Minor problems in the feet usually respond to a Dr. Scholl's "610" which you can buy at a Dr. Scholl's shoe store. If the heel lift is needed, a half-inch or less of surgical felt will most often do the trick.

Q: I also have weak abdominals, and tight back, hamstring and calf muscles. What do I do about that?

A: Since the main reason for low-back pain is weak abdominal muscles, the heart of the treatment is in correcting them. The most effective exercises are bent-leg situps with the back flat against the floor and Kendall's isometric lumbar flexion exercises. Flexibility difficulties will respond to wall pushups, hamstring stretching and the backover—lying flat on the floor and bringing your legs with the knees locked to touch the floor behind your head.

Q: What are the Kendall exercises?

A: Contract your abdominal muscles as hard as possible, pulling your navel toward your spine. Relax. Contract your seat or buttocks muscles as hard as you can. Relax. Do both together. Hold each for 15 seconds. Repeat 15 times, as often as you think of it during the day. The exercise can be done at any time, while walking, sitting or even driving a car.

Q: What about manipulation?

A: Manipulation is a valuable initial therapy. It frequently gets the patient back into alignment, which then can be maintained by the procedures already outlined. Unfortunately, it is either never used or is overused. Nevertheless, it has a definite place in the treatment of low-back problems.

Q: Any final words?

A: Continue running or playing your sport. Avoid speed work and hill running. Avoid straight-leg situps; they can cause back trouble. Do your exercises before and after each training session. Remember, you control the situation. You have a special susceptibility to this problem. Only by diligence and perseverance in your exercises and the other measures can you avoid recurrences.

BACK EXERCISES

Q: I am a 51-year-old who has always been an active sportsman. For the past five years, I have been doing long-distance running and have run the 56-mile Comrades Marathon three times.

My problem is my back. At times, it has been so bad I have

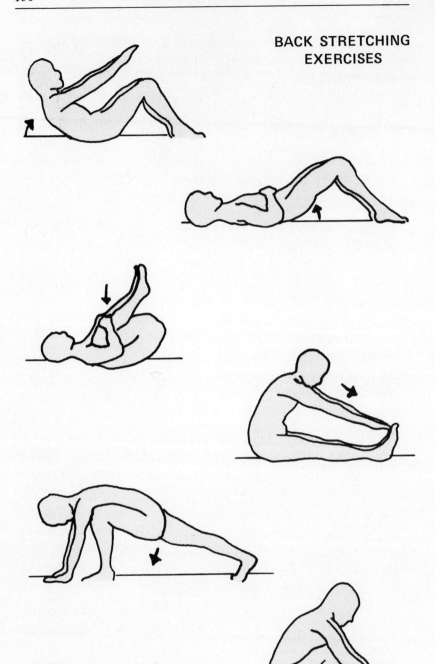

Abdominal muscle exercises help
keep the spine in line

had to crawl off the bed onto the floor and then slowly onto my feet. My X-rays show a slippage of the spine.

Since the last Comrades, I have been in constant trouble. I feel all right while running, but am sore that night and the following day. I have tried everything except stopping running. What should I do?

A: By all means, do not stop running. It is not the actual running but the side-effects of it that are bothering you. It is the muscle imbalance you develop in running that stresses your back.

The answer is to balance your muscles. Stretch the muscles overdeveloped by the running. Strengthen those which are being overpowered by the strong tight muscles.

Stretch the gastrocs, hamstrings and iliopsoas by doing the backover. Do this before and after running for at least 5-10 minutes.

Next, strengthen your glutei and belly muscles so they will straighten out your spine. Lie on your back with your knees bent. Tighten your buttocks muscles and come up to a sitting position. Do as many as you can up to 20 after each workout.

Q: You have stated that bent-leg situps are a remedy for sciatic pain. My question is, when you say "remedy," do you mean that a runner should wait until he gets sciatic pain to do the situps, or should they be done by all runners as a preventive?

A: Runners should do bent-leg situps as part of their daily routine. Along with flexibility exercises, they will help prevent sciatic pain. In addition, the number of bent-leg situps you can do correlates with resistance to exhaustion.

Unfortunately, we runners are lazy. We will do any amount of mileage, which we love, but will find reasons to skip our exercises.

Q: I was doing one of your Magic Six exercises, the backover, and, much to my chagrin, I got an excruciating pain in my lower back. I attempted to run with this and my efforts failed.

Since that time, the pain has traveled to my hip. I not only can't run, but also get shots of pain when I cough and when I urinate and defecate. I have done some individual research on the matter, and I am guessing that it has to do with the sciatic nerve with depressingly suspicious sounds of a slipped disc. I have a doctor's appointment in the near future, but, typical of their antagonistic attitude towards distance running, I expect a prescription of non-activity. I would like your opinion on the matter.

A: The road back will depend not on flexibility of the spine (if only because these exercises bother you). It will depend on developing strength in the abdominals. You have definite sciatic nerve irritation and have either ruptured a disc or caused further slippage.

Keep up your conditioning for two or three weeks with cycling or swimming, and do bent-leg situps as your major exercise.

I had a similar experience almost 10 years ago while doing interval 300-yard dashes. On the 12th or 13th one, I got the pain but refused to stop. I weathered a three-week siege, but still get back and sciatic pain if I neglect my exercises.

"POTHOLE STRAIN"

Q: One morning, I accidentally stepped into a pothole while running alongside a highway. Nearly falling, I felt a slight pain in my leg but was able to continue to run. The next day, however, my thigh hurt as though a muscle had been pulled. I couldn't run without limping, and I developed a pain in the area of the hip on the other leg. Three months later, the pain in the hip persists.

A: Apparently your limp, whatever the cause, created a strain in your spinal-pelvic junction, which is causing your hip pain. This pain, therefore, is "referred pain." That is to say, pain carried along a nerve from your now maladjusted spine to your hip area.

If I am right, you will have to start on exercises to correct this lack of alignment. Stretch your hamstrings and iliopsoas to allow flattening of the back. And do abdominal situps to strenghen your abdominal muscles. In addition, I would recom-

mend the use of a lumbo-sacral belt made by Bellhorn or
Futuro.

These measures may take time. Do not be discouraged.

Chapter 20
General Wear and Tear

POUND FOOLISH?

Q: I recently read an article mentioning that "the problem with exercise is that it plays hell with one's knees and ankles." It mentioned the damage pro basketball players do to their knees with the constant pounding, and stated that "what is not so clear is the long term effect of jogging on the knees and ankles."

What is the effect of running 5-10 miles per day, about six days per week, on the knees and ankles? Is there really a lack of information on this subject? I enjoy running on a recreational basis and to stay in shape. But if I am going to incur permanent damage in the process, I think I might be wise to switch to bicycling.

A: I saw that article, and it upset me because it reflected again the ignorance of what a sports podiatrist can do for the knee and ankle. Maintaining the neutral position of the foot through footstrike and takeoff can give you injury-free mileage for the rest of your life.

Your body tells you when such help is necessary. That is what pain is for: to prevent you from injuring yourself. If you are running with pain, you should see to your shoes, exercises, and advice from a sports podiatrist. If you are running pain-free, you can thumb your nose at whoever wrote that article.

Progressive damage to joints and deterioration from running

is one of those theories that "stands to reason that it should be this way." Actually, few things stand to reason, and hardly anything in relation to the human body.

The garden-variety human body is capable of long-term, trouble-free use if properly cared for. We are born with a 70-year warranty, and it will stand up if we don't abuse it.

Dr. Ernst van Aaken, a strong figure in veterans' running in Europe, would laugh at such contentions of damage from use, as would the Tarahumara Indians of Mexico who go through life on their legs and feet.

Nietzsche once wrote that any thought arrived at while sitting down should be suspect. This seems to be one of them. The problems runners get into are due to structural or postural instability. Correction of these problems will give any runner the mileage potential of a Rolls Royce.

ARTHRITIS

Q: Do you have any information concerning the breakdown of joints, specifically the hip and knee joints of individuals who have been running for many years?

A: Although many middle-aged runners have been told by their physicians that arthritis will occur, there is no scientific evidence to substantiate this.

One study done in England, where hip arthritis is much more prevalent than in the U.S., suggested running as a factor. Those who had compulsory running as school boys had more arthritis than those who weren't required to run.

I question these conclusions. Schoolboy running occurs in the formative years, and where significant foot abnormalities are present (they did not study this) and running was not taken up naturally, I could see damage to a hip joint.

This should not indict prolonged distance running in someone who has fused his bones, takes to running naturally and is able — with or without foot supports — to run pain-free. When these conditions exist, your knees and hips should handle any mileage.

Otto Appenzeller, M.D., adds to my comments on arthritis in

runners. Appenzeller is associated with the University of New Mexico Medical School:

Myths abound about the ill effects of running. Among others, there is a widespread belief that physical strain on joints during running may lead in later years to osteoarthritis.

A recent paper reviewed the hip joints of 74 former runners of Finnish descent. Each of the subjects had won a championship, and almost all had at one time or another held a Finnish record. Some achieved world-record times. When the joints were examined by x-rays, the average age of the athletes was 65 years, and they had started training at an average age of 15 (range 12-25). They participated in competitive running for a mean 21 years (range 8-50). One hundred fifteen male patients from a hospital were used as controls. None of them had been admitted because of hip complaints, and the x-rays of the hips were done for other purposes. The age distribution in this non-athletic control group was similar to that of the runners (mean 56, range 40-75).

This study showed that osteoarthritis was found in only 4% of the athletes but in 8.7% of the controls. Competitive running, therefore, cannot be considered a contributing factor to arthritis of hip. The cause of osteoarthritis remains a mystery, but this study excludes the possibility that physical strain which might occur while running contributes to the development of arthritis.

It is, of course, not surprising that running should in fact protect hip joints from arthritis, for the hip is designed for walking and running. It also needs to be recognized that motion is necessary for nutrition of the various components of the joint. Intermittent pressure apparently allows the joint fluid to circulate in very much the same way as air enters the lungs during alternate squeezing and release. Prolonged immobility or continuous pressure has been shown to damage the joint surfaces.

It seems that in the human body tissues are adapted to their normal function. If normal function is denied them, as is the case in "normal" Western society, degeneration of structures is, if not induced, at least hastened.

HIP PAIN

Q: I run 50-60 miles per week and have completed my first marathon. My problem is a sharp pain in my right hip. It is at the top of the hip bone, and is tender to the touch and painful while running. What should I do?

A: Troubles up to and including the knee usually are due to a combination of (1) weak feet; (2) muscle imbalance; (3) wrong shoes. Usually, help comes quickly.

With hip pain, however, things get sticky. The foot may be a factor but only in perhaps one-third of the cases. Even the local diagnosis is difficult. Runners are told they have arthritis, bursitis, tendinitis, neuritis. Even the structure involved may not be identified.

So hip pain means a complete systems analysis. Hunt out every abnormality and treat it:

1. Weak feet, particularly high-arched feet.

2. Leg-length discrepancy, a freqent cause of hip and sciatic pain.

3. Tight hamstrings and weak abdominals. Use of the back-over exercise and bent-leg situps is essential.

4. Overstriding and other errors in form must be corrected. Avoid racing and hill work until you get a diagnosis and finally a cure.

BONE STRESS

Q: It is the opinion of Eric Rodin, M.D., that stress fractures and joint damage are due to fatigued muscles. Instead of absorbing the shock, they pass the job on to the bone. The message, therefore, is beware of taxing long runs. Far better to divy up that mileage into a number of workouts. I send you Dr. Rodin's study.

A: You're most likely right. When the muscles fatigue, things begin to go awry. Shock is magnified, and the evidence is that this involves the knee and the hip.

However, I do not think this sort of fatigue occurs due to distance. It is more likely to occur with daily running and inadequate recovery between runs.

Approaching a training run with zest (usually a matter of 1-3 days rest between) assures me of a pleasant 80-90 minutes of running. I am unaware of any shock problems and frequently feel at my best toward the end of the run.

We may both be right. Stress fractures occur in weaker bones, but they also occur at the point of greatest stress (the stress fracture of the second metatarsal in Morton's foot, for example.

Wear and tear is not answer enough. There has to be an individual susceptibility, some biomechanical mischief.

The solution? Correct shoes (still a chancy thing); daily and prolonged exercises for strength/flexibility balance; arch supports either to control the footstrike or to increase the weight-bearing area.

Stop running or go to those mini-distances? Never. Dr. Rodin suggests that joint degeneration is not a disease but the end result of poorly handled mechanical loading. We seem to be saying the same thing. His shock absorber is the muscles; mine is primarily the foot, secondarily the muscles.

PUBIC BONE FRACTURE

Q: I visited a running clinic for continued groin discomfort, went the usual orthopedic-and-exercise route, but still had no luck. Eventually it took a bone scan to detect a stress fracture in the public bone region. I was told this happens very rarely.

A: Persistent groin pain is one of the most difficult problems a runner can encounter. When someone writes to me with that symptom, I know instantly my reply is going to be unsatisfactory. Over the past few years, I have suggested all types of therapy, almost all proving unsuccessful.

One reason is just what occurred with you, a stress fracture. I am inclined to believe that they are nowhere near as rare as we are told. X-rays are taken too early or not at all. Even in the best hands, stress fractures can be missed. Frequently, as with you, a bone scan must be done. This is expensive and therefore infrequent procedure.

Nevertheless, after muscle inbalance and leg-length discrepancies have been corrected and unusual sciatic syndromes have been ruled out, a stress fracture should be looked for. Women may be particularly susceptible to this overuse syndrome.

The treatment is six weeks away from running. After that, running can be resumed, but a diligent search should be made to correct the basic cause. This may be:

1. *Shoes with poor shock absorption.* Could undercut heels contribute to this? I don't think anyone knows. Certainly, the flanges on the heels increase shock.

2. *Poor form.* Overstriding and bouncing, increasing shock on impact.

3. *Too rigid feet.* Most feet have to be controlled and movement prevented. In rigid feet, however, movement becomes necessary. One runner I know got help unwittingly by reversing his supports, putting the right one in the left shoe and vice versa, thus creating movement rather than controlling it.

4. *Muscle rigidity and inflexibility.* Muscles maintain balance. When they are either weak or inflexible, impact shock increases.

5. *Factor "X."* The question when a person gets an overuse illness is "why me? How am I different from other runners who wear the same shoes, do the same mileage, etc." It's a puzzlement.

BOW LEGS

Q: For the past five years, I have coached a college cross-country team and during that time have had several runners whose legs bow out. Without exception, they have experienced knee problems at one time or another. This usually occurs when the weekly mileage climbs to 70 or individuals runs exceed 15 miles. Could a different footplant help?

A: A different footplant, more pigeon-toed, is desirable in a lot of foot-leg-knee problems but is rarely obtained. Runners fall into the normal gait dicated by their structure.

Bow legs cause a marked reaction at footstrike which is transmitted to the knee. This can be a difficult problem, but a corrective insert in the shoe (an inside wedge) can be helpful.

TRY WALKING

Q: Because running causes pain to my lower back and knees, I'd like to investigate race walking.

A: You sound like an exceptionally fine prospect for race walking. Runners with low-back pain and intractable knee problems have found a pain-free haven in the walking sport. The improvement in knee injuries is easily explained. The obligatory locked knee at footstrike keeps the patella in its grove. The usual wandering of the kneecap is thus prevented.

Why the low-back difficulties are benefitted are not quite so clear. Again, it probably relates to the mechanics. Good footstrike, locked knee, flattening of the spine—all contribute.

PART FIVE:
CARDIOVASCULAR SYSTEM

*"There is no disease that needs more advice
and less medicine than heart disease."*

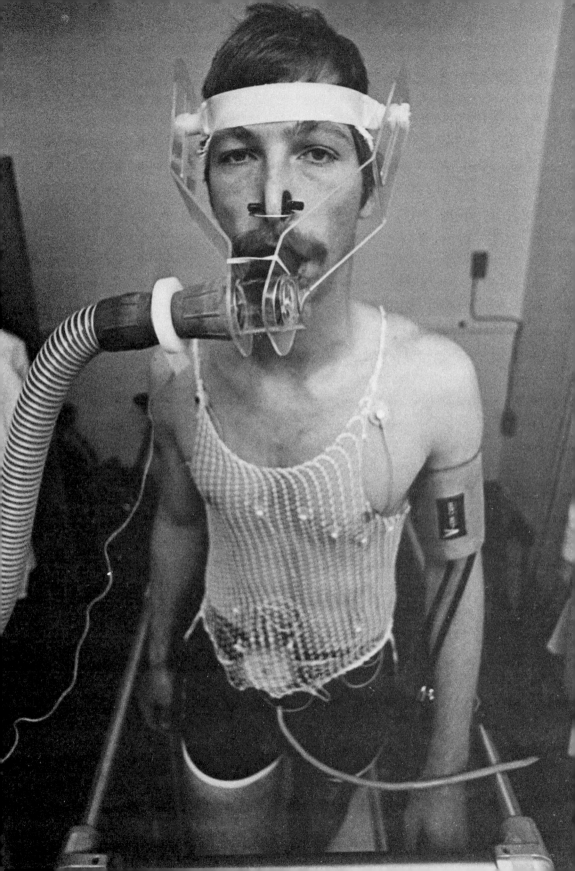

Chapter 21
Getting to the Heart

Is running safe? If so, why do we continually read newspaper reports of people collapsing and dying while out running? If not, how can we make it safe?

These questions are being raised continually, if not by runners and potential runners, then by cardiologists who either support or oppose running as a means to physical fitness. These experts disagree on results as well as safety. Some, for instance, see running as ineffective as well as dangerous. Dr. Meyer Friedman, who first described the Type A personality syndrome, states that any male over 35 should restrict his exercise activity to billiards or croquet.

Others who spend their lives conducting cardiac rehabilitation programs say it is the most effective way to achieve fitness and protection from heart attacks. Their views have been reinforced by Dr. Ralph Paffenbarger's study on Harvard graduates. He discovered significant reduction in coronary disease when the individual did vigorous exercise amounting to 2000 calories a week.

As for safety, there is one fact that most experts agree upon. Sudden deaths do not occur in persons with a healthy heart. Dr. Ernst Jokl, in his book *Exercise and Cardiac Death*, states: "Not one instance was encountered in which death could be regarded as due to the effects of extreme exertion on a previously healthy heart."

How, then, to prove your heart is health? Suggestions range

from "listen to your body" all the way up to a stress test. For Dr. Friedman, even the stress tests are not enough. They are, he claims, too unreliable. They say there is heart disease when there is none, and they say there is no heart disease where there is.

According to Dr. Friedman, X-rays are the only sure way to know the condition of your coronary arteries, which is true. X-rays are the Supreme Court. They are also expensive and dangerous.

My own feelings are mixed. I would acknowledge the danger. Crossing the street can be dangerous if you are daydreaming. We learn to live defensively as we learn to drive defensively. Nature will always give us a warning, but we must be listening.

From a study of a number of sudden deaths while running it was discovered that over one half of the runners had mentioned some warning symptoms either to a doctor or a spouse. These warnings weren't heeded.

I also see the danger as relative to a person. There are favored people who, running or not, have a statistical resistance to coronary disease. They are doomed to some death other than a heart attack. They can run with impunity, knowing that no matter how they abuse their cardiopulminary system, it will never fail them. When I die, they will have to take my heart out and beat it to death with a stick.

There are others, however, who must approach running with a lot more intelligence then I do. They are statistically more susceptible to attacks and more likely to be harboring asymptomatic disease.

A study of 5000 coronary deaths in New York City found a predominance of endo-mesomorphs. These are people with big frames and a tendency toward overweight. Such people are, for the most part, aggressive, energetic, ambitious individuals who embody the characteristics of Friedman's Type A personality. They tend to attack their fitness program with the same intensity they do their work. In such instances, fatalities can occur even in closely supervised rehabilitation programs. Dr. Terence Kavanagh in Toronto, an outstanding figure in this field, has reported deaths in patients who were determined to improve their mile times every time they got out on the track.

Exercise can, of course, be dangerous. We have only to read papers after each snowfall to be convinced of that. Paul Dudley

White, a proponent of vigorous exercise, used to begin his lecture with a headline from the *Boston Globe* that stated in large type the number of deaths in the Boston area from shoveling snow.

Running, however, is a completely different body maneuver. In running, the degree of effort is determined solely by the runner. There is no need to strain or get short of breath, two things that occur while shoveling snow. Nor does the opponent control the pace of the activity, as can happen in tennis, basketball and other sports.

The oddity is that if something is wrong with your coronary tree, running is probably the best medicine there is. There is even more reason to be in an exercise program than not.

I was in a race with 7000 people in Chicago. I doubt if more than a handful had taken their stress tests. I would be surprised if any had gone through angiography of their coronary vessels. They have already decided. They are going back to those primitive days when life depended on being fit and are learning the ancient ways of doing it.

There is no substitute for learning to live in our bodies. All the tests and all the machines in the world will fail if we do not first become good animals.

Chapter 22
Reading the Responses

"ABNORMAL" EKG

The EKG machine's potential for interfering in an athlete's life was predicted from the work of Venerando and Rulli at the Rome Olympics.

The Italians studied a group of 89 world-class marathoners and 38 walkers, and found abnormalities (by current opinion) in almost all of them. Fully 12% had negative T-waves in the leads taken over the chest wall, a finding previously considered indicative of serious disease. More than 50% had abnormal conduction between the ventricles, and 15% had abnormally high electrical voltage. There were numerous other but less forbidding changes on the graphs.

The Venerando report suggested that any routine EKG screening of endurance athletes would turn up a number of odd and disturbing EKG tracings, and almost all these records could bother the usual electrocardiographer.

The prediction has come true, mostly because this report (along with another from Israel) has not reached general acceptance. It is difficult, you see, to conceive that changes usually connected with disease can occur in a heightened physiological state—which endurance fitness is.

Runners subjecting themselves to comprehensive physical examination (my advice is to get one for a baseline and then see a doctor only when you are sick) should be aware that their

EKG may be misinterpreted.

It is well to remember Venerando's conclusions: The changes are not related to decreased heart function or disease; they are not accompanied by any heart enlargement beyond that physiological change associated with the sport.

Similar "normal abnormalities" have been reported with other groups of athletes:

• *Heart "murmur"*—A test of one group of college lacrosse players indicated that 11 of 15 athletes had a "third sound" after exercising. Researcher Dave Lavine said the third sound is often thought to be indicative of heart disease, but "before being studied, the heart of each player was given a thorough cardiological examination. All had sound hearts. The murmurs developed *after* the hearts were well conditioned. At resting stage, a well-conditioned heart will pump more blood at a slower rate than normal, thus producing the murmur-type sound. Once an athlete is out of training, the murmur and sounds should disappear."

Lavine noted that doctors should recognize the "third sound" as a healthy one, and not to diagnose it improperly as a heart problem.

• *Palpitations or irregular pulse*—Irregular pulse and premature heart beats are rarely indicative of heart disease. They are usually due to constitutional disease such as thyroid, allergy or excessive use of stimulants. They are sometimes seen as an exhaustion symptom. Runners might do well to taper off training when they occur.

• *Slow pulse*—Most runners are "vagotonic." Their vagus nerve which slows the pulse (as well as narrowing the pupils and increasing stomach acid secretions) is dominant. Slow pulse, down in the 50s, 40s or even lower, is common and no cause for concern.

• *Low blood pressure*—Of itself, it is no problem. But if blood pressure falls when a person stands, light-headedness or even fainting may occur. This state frequently is experienced when an athlete is training heavily. It is felt, like so many other unusual body signs, to be an exhaustion phenomenon and may mean the runner is at or passing his peak.

"ABNORMAL" PULSE

Q: For 25 years or more, my heart beat has been slow—60, more or less. But in the last couple of years, when I've been running seriously, it has been in the 50s and 40s. At the Red Cross Bloodmobile, I was tested in the mid-40s. The attending doctor rejected me as a donor. I argued that low heart rate was a sign of health, but he rejoined, "not that low," and "with reduced pressure after donating blood you might get a heart block." What do you think?

A: Your pulse and mine are identical. Such a rate is quite common among athletes, especially distance runners. The pulse rate is no reason not to give blood, and most knowledgeable physicians would give you a quick okay.

Q: At a party recently, a medical student bet me his car that he could not test my heart beat under 50 per minute. Since I have started running, my heart beat has dropped considerably and I have tested it at about 42 when awakening in the morning. He claims I would be in a comatose state at anything under 50 and that I must be too sleepy to count correctly. What are my chances of winning his car?

A: You have already won your bet, since fit runners routinely have pulses below 50. It appears that the current crop of physicians may graduate with the same ignorance of exercise physiology that I had when I received my M.D. It has come to the point that we runners are teaching the physicians rather than the other way around.

HIGH PULSE RATE

Q: Though I train fairly hard, I cannot get my basal pulse rate much below the low 60s, while my contemporaries (with similar times) have theirs in the 40s. However, my maximum pulse rate is 240-plus, well above everyone else's. I had thought I was at least moderately fit, but the pulse rate seems to indicate otherwise. Am I just not training hard enough?

A: Too much is made of resting pulse. Roger Bannister's was 38 when he broke the four-minute barrier, but Jim Ryun's was 72 when he ran the mile more than eight seconds faster. Studies of Olympic marathoners revealed a basal heart rate ranging from 50-76.

Each individual has an optimum basal rate. At this rate, his body is in a state of overall fitness. His various body systems are in harmony. He is, you could say, in tune. This rate is probably controlled by the autonomic nervous system.

Performance, however, is much more related to exercise and post-exercise heart rates. Stroke volume (the amount of blood ejected with each beat) is one of the big differentials between a superstar and an ordinary runner. A maximum oxygen uptake test would give a much better picture of what you can do than your resting pulse.

PEAK PULSE

Q: After a long series of running injuries, frustrations and failures, my communards and I finally discovered the sense and security of aerobic running. All the while, I had been under the impression that this aerobic pace involved pulses ranging from 130-150 beats per minute, with 160 as an outside figure.

On a recent six-mile run, however, we timed our pulses and the results were unnerving. After about a mile, our first reading gave me a pulse of about 150 and the last reading after the sixth mile a 180. Now, what puzzles me is that at no time did I even approach breathlessness. So what goes on here? Is 180 a notable reading for a slow pace? What about the lack of any correlation between pulse and breathing?

A: Maximal pulse rate is the key to the solution of your problem. When you know this and know at what percent of your aerobic capacity you are working, your pulse should be explained.

Maximal pulse decreases with age. Mine is 180. When I go through an easy six-mile workout, my pulse when I re-enter my office or kitchen is about 140.

If age isn't the answer, I would suppose you are running at the top of your aerobic capacity.

POST-RUN PULSE

Q: How long should it take a heartbeat to return to normal after a run?

A: As a rule of thumb, your pulse should come down below 100 within 10 minutes. It usually will in five. From then on, progress can be slow. In 15 minutes, it may return to 10 points above your basal pulse. At top shape, it will probably be basal by that time.

All-out, exhausting efforts, especially those that may put you past that fine line of fitness, are followed by prolonged elevation. Once, after running the Boston Marathon on Monday, I ran a Masters mile at the Penn Relays on Saturday. Six hours later, my pulse was still 110. I didn't run another good race for six weeks.

MEASURING PULSE

Q: Some engineer friends of mine have developed a device to measure and display pulse rate while running. We think it will help beginning runners to "train, not strain" by maintaining their pulse at 60-80% of their maximum rate. It will also show premature beats and other cardiac irregularities. Do you think it would be helpful?

A: I have led the fight to free athletes, especially runners, from such devices. Mine has been a campaign to listen to your body. I'm not saying this wouldn't be an excellent research tool for those people who direct cardiac rehabilitation programs. But "train, don't strain" implies we should use our body's reactions to effort rather than setting running pace to the desired heart rate.

IRREGULAR PULSE

Q: Would you please discuss arrythmias? What are they, what causes them, what effect they have on one's health, and how common they are?

A: Cardiac arrythmias are disorders of the heart beat and are usually described as palpitations of the heart. They can vary from simple premature beats felt as something flopping over in the chest to long, continued runs of extremely rapid beats.

The majority of arrythmias occur in healthy hearts and have no effect on general health. The heart muscle can initiate its own beat, and this is therefore an exaggeration of a normal property. Some people seem to have a tendency to arrythmias and have them under severe stress.

Abnormal conduction of the pulse waves through the heart apparently makes an individual more susceptible. I have such a condition, known as Wolff-Parkinson-White syndrome. Tension and speedwork without warmup can make my pulse very irregular. I also note some skipping or missing of the pulse at the wrist when overtraining. This occurs when the beat comes too soon and before the heart fills, so no pulse wave is initiated.

I believe such benign irregularities are common among runners, ordinary as well as world-class.

SILENT ATTACK

Q: After over 25 years of enjoying distance running, I was recently informed that an at-rest electrocardiogram indicated I have, at some time between early childhood and not too recently, had a "silent myocardial infarction of the left ventricle"—a heart attack. Poised at the beginning of my Masters career, this came as a most ironic and traumatic bit of news. After the tests, the doctor said he was not a bit concerned. But I'd like to find out what the complete story might be so as to at least set my mind at rest, if not to revise my training and goals. Have you ever heard of a comparable case?

A: I'm encouraged by your physician's approach to your difficulty. It suggests that your overall examination is excellent. That leaves us with explaining and dealing with the EKG. Several possibilities come to mind:

First, you may have an "abnormal normal EKG." One summer, I did EKGs on an entire professional football squad and saw readings that could easily be read as heart attacks. Further examination, however, indicated that there was no damage or threat of trouble.

Second, you may have had some inflammation of the heart when younger which left you with some EKG abnormality of no clinical significance.

Finally, it is remotely possible that you had a coronary. But I doubt it. In any case, I guess an exercise stress test would clear the air and ease your mind.

CHEST PAINS

Q: In 30 days, I lost 40 pounds. Later, I started running. The second day, after three-fourths of a mile, I had a pain in the center of my chest. It happened again three weeks later, during a three-mile run. A doctor gave me a thorough examination and said nothing was wrong with my heart. Can you tell me why I've been having these pains, and whether or not it is safe to continue running?

A: Pain in the center of the chest brought on by exertion and relieved by rest is something you must treat with respect. Even with normal EKGs and normal blood chemistry, it could represent heart disease.

I suggest that this pain is a red light in your exercise program. Establish a perimeter of distance and speed that causes such difficulty, then stay within it. This may mean that you will be restricted to 30 minutes of walking on an empty stomach once a day. This should be done at a pace your body recognizes as minimal to mild exertion.

After three months of that, I suggest you have a stress test to evaluate your heart circulation and your fitness.

HEART INFLAMMATION

Q: A friend started feeling weak during runs. (He is 48 years old and normally runs 7-11 miles daily.) Along with the weakness, he had a shortness of breath. Finally, he went in for a physical and was hospitalized, as his resting pulse rate was 144. He was given eight shock treatments in two days to try to lower the pulse, but this failed.

He was sent to the Cleveland Clinic to undergo treatment, hoping to determine the problem. They told him that the lining of his heart was weak and would not strengthen. If the problem is with the myocardium, as he was told, isn't that muscle and won't muscle strengthen? He was told "no heavy exercise" and to find easier work (he installed telephones).

Can you give us any hope, or is the doctor right in saying he won't be able to run again?

A: I have reviewed the disquieting report on your friend. I have searched it for something optimistic to say and possibly will. But at first glance, it appears that he developed some inflammation of the heart muscle, had an episode of almost intractable fibrillation and is now in a quiescent but weakened state.

Primary myocardial disease is a large area. It can be because of alcohol or infection or unknown causes. Its effects also vary from complete incapacity to mild disability.

My own feeling is that improvement should occur over a period of 3-6 months. In addition, I find it very favorable that his heart size is not enlarged and, although ventricular impairment is present, he is in no failure.

I think the question is when he can run and how fast. I would start with a brisk walking program. Then, move on to a slow run every other day. This should be done at mild exertion, being sure he can talk with a running companion. It would be nice to have a stress test done and see his pulse response before running is started.

However, I would hold this off until about 8-10 weeks of 30 minutes brisk walking four days a week.

HOW SAFE IS IT?

Q: I am aware of the values of exercise on the average person, and I know running programs are often used for cardiac patients. My question is, at what point is a person's condition too serious to be helped by exercise? My father has a heart murmur and circulatory problems caused by atherosclerosis. He is 58.

A: There is no disease that needs more advice and less medicine than heart disease. And the advice I give to my patients is to become an athlete, albeit a limited one.

People understand about athletes. They know they warm up before they compete; that they wait until their food is digested before they become active; that they avoid alcohol and tobacco and anything else that would interfere with maximum performance; that they want to be just bone and muscle.

But first of all, they must find their sport. Cardiacs who become athletes have to pick from low-grade endurance sports: cycling, walking, jogging, golfing, perhaps doubles tennis.

In your father's instance, I would advise walking. Unless he has previously been in those other sports, they will be too strenuous—at least at the start. After a period of time on a walking program, reaching 1-1½ miles in 30 minutes four times a week, he can move into other activities should he wish to do so.

DOUBLE DEATH

Q: I recently read of two runners both collapsing and dying during the same run. This makes a 54-year-old runner like myself wary. Have you heard of this tragedy.

A: The death of two men running together is enough to unsettle anyone. Apparently, the 48-year-old man collapsed first, and when the 61-year-old ran for help he also collapsed. They died within five minutes of each other at the hospital.

Unfortunately, after such reports in the paper we seldom get any further details. Most of these incidents occur in random fashion, are casually investigated by the coroner (since coroners are primarily concerned with foul play), and life goes on. Nothing is learned.

Several questions weren't answered: Were they experiencing chest pain with exertion? Had they been pushing to improve their time? Was there a bad family history of coronary artery disease? Any coexistent diabetes or hypertension? Why running and not walking? What were the personalities of the two men? Were they Type-A personality people attacking a fitness program?

From investigations into the sudden-death syndrome, it appears that about 80% are "electrical" deaths, so-called ventricular fibrillation. They are not due to acute heart damage, i.e., acute myocardial infarction.

Ventricular fibrillation can occur anytime but probably can also be initiated by excitement or strenuous exertion—for instance, at a race track or while shoveling snow.

Even in the best-regulated cardiac rehabilitation programs, collapse occasionally occurs. My feeling is that most of us are blind and deaf tenants of our bodies. If you really listen to your body, you don't need professional help. If you don't listen, all the supervision and testing isn't going to protect you.

In the final analysis, we don't know if this incident was predictable and preventable. I wish someone would tell us what's going on.

Q: Would you please comment on an article in the September 1975 issue of *Moneysworth* ("Joggers Get Physically Fit for a Fatal Coronary") which says, in part, "Despite the claims of many physicians and hordes of thundering faddists, little or no proof exists that strenuous exercise does anything to delay or prevent disease."

A: I haven't prepared a full-dress response to the anti-runner because I think they have their truth just as we have our truth. But I am not going to listen to anyone suggesting that what is an integral part of my life, something that has shown me who I am, can be dangerous or detrimental.

On the other hand, something must be said to keep others who are runners to the very core of their being from giving up or never trying this life-supporting activity.

Articles like the one in *Moneysworth* are aimed at those people who don't listen to their bodies and try to change them too fast. They attack nature rather than cooperate with it.

Chapter 23
It's in the Blood

HIGH BLOOD PRESSURE

The doctors are at it again. In their endless desire to give us healthier and happier and longer lives, they have turned their attention to high blood pressure. We are now seeing the birth of a new and major phenomenon in American medicine, the hypertension industry.

Not only physicians but members of allied health professions have joined in this project. It has become almost impossible to avoid having your blood pressure taken, if not in a doctor's office, then in a shopping mall.

Once your blood pressure is taken and found to be elevated, there is a good chance that your life will be substantially changed, if not by the side-effects of medication, then by worry. The big weapon in any campaign of this kind is the scare approach—not how good you are going to feel but how bad things are going to get.

What is the truth of this mixture of threats and promises? We might well quote from an editor in the *British Medical Journal*: "In no other division of medicine is opinion more confused than in that which deals with the cause and significance of blood pressure, and the progress and treatment of any patient that may exhibit it."

The truth is that doctors are dragging their feet as much as are their patients. The physicians, particularly the older and

162

more experienced ones, seem to have no more interest in prescribing medications for blood pressure than the patients have
for taking them.

Many older doctors agree with psychiatrist Viktor Frankl, "If
I measure the blood pressure of a patient, find it slightly increased and then tell the patient about it, I actually do not tell
him the truth," Frankl explains, "for he will become more nervous, and the blood pressure will increase more. If I tell him in
reverse, that he need not worry, I do not tell him a lie, for he
will be calmed down, and his blood pressure will become
normal."

Sir George Pickering, probably the world's foremost investi-
gator into the clinical manifestations of high blood pressure,
takes much the same point of view. "Never frighten the patient" is Pickering's dictum.

Not only do physicians frighten patients, but they do it un-
necessarily. "One extremely inconvenient fact," states Pickering, is that blood pressure bounces around during the day. It
can go from 60 over 30 while you are asleep up to 160 over 100
while you are making love.

There are, as Frankl and Pickering point out, patients whose
blood pressure is only up when it is being taken. You cannot get
the cuff on fast enough to obtain a normal reading. The
adrenalin is already in the system and working. The natural
response to stress, only to an abnormal degree, is already in
operation.

"In prescribing medication for such a patient," writes Dr.
Mark Altschule of Harvard, "the physician is treating himself
rather than the patient."

Such an opinion is also supported by Dr. Milton Mendelowitz
of Mount Sinai Medical School: "Such hypertensive patients,
particularly those with transient or early stress hypertension,
should not be treated at all."

How can one establish this type of blood pressure and the
fact that there is no need to treat it? One method that I have
discovered is have the person hyperventilate. This, however, has
to be surreptitious.

If the patient is aware of the purpose of the hyperventilation,
the resultant tension is enough to maintain the elevation of the

blood pressure. I usually pretend to be listening to the lungs and instruct the patient to take long, slow, deep breaths again and again. Eventually, the relaxation comes. Then, I sneak around, pump up the cuff, and *Voila!*, a normal pressure.

The idea, you see, is to turn off the brain, to prevent the perception of stress to interfere, to eliminate worry and fear and tension and anger, and thereby get to a baseline reading.

So transient blood pressure needs no treatment. But what about a fixed elevated blood pressure? At what level should that be treated?

The first thing to do with high blood pressure is to define it. It is not a disease; it is a risk factor. When present, it makes it more likely that you will develop either heart or kidney disease, or a stroke. In this, it is much the same as smoking, obesity and high cholesterol—risk factors all.

These items can be measured, and in their magnitude establish greater or lesser risk. So can blood pressure. What, then, is the normal range? At what point is blood pressure high? When must treatment be instituted?

Sir George Pickering has repeatedly challenged every medical audience he has addressed in the past 25 years to provide a fixed dividing line between normal blood pressure and hypertension. Hypertension, it appears, is in the eyes of the beholder. One person's hypertension is normal pressure to someone else. What is permissible in some clinics is cause for treatment in others. Agreement generally occurs when the level reaches 170 over 110. Below this, however, the argument still rages.

Whatever the level, many experts now agree that it is better to follow the patient for a while rather than institute immediate treatment. Large studies have shown that blood pressures of 160 over 100 show no progression in fully 80% of individuals followed without treatment over the years.

Many of these are undoubtedly members of that large group whose blood pressure is only up when it is taken. The tipoff to this is an incidental hospitalization where blood pressure readings become a matter of course and don't upset the patient. If surgery has been done, then the pressure under general anesthesia also provides the baseline reading for a patient.

The decision to initiate treatment should also take into account evidence, or lack of it, that the blood pressure is affecting the body. A normal EKG, normal chest plates and negative urine examinations should indicate to the physician that the blood pressure is still a number and not a disease.

But even if treatment be deemed necessary, that treatment should be tailored to the patient. Hypertension is an indication of a susceptible individual living in a stressful situation who is unable to cope.

We now know that one of these genetic susceptibilities is the inability to handle salt. In saltless societies, there is no hypertension. In societies with a heavy salt intake, like ours, hypertension abounds.

Obesity, another factor, also unfortunately abounds. So the first thing a hypertensive must do is limit salt and get down to a lean weight. For most people, that would be what they weighed at college graduation or on their wedding day.

Patients with high blood pressure cannot handle salt. They cannot handle being overweight. And they cannot handle their present lifestyle, their way of being in the world. High blood pressure, like drinking and smoking and nail biting, is an indication that the job or the family or the people around are arousing fear and frustration instead of bringing happiness and joy.

There are two ways to deal with this. One way is to eliminate the stress. The other is to increase the ability to cope with it.

Coping depends on self-image, physical, spiritual and mental fitness, and a sense of humor. None of these is available on prescription. They have to be fought for and earned—a big package to ask from an individual who can also get a normal blood pressure simply by taking three pills a day. Still, in the long run, it is the only way to go. The patient with a blood pressure problem must realize that his problem is a lifestyle problem.

You will notice I have said nothing about drugs. I won't, except to warn against them. If nothing else, they fix the person in the problem. They remove the patient's responsibility, the need for effort, discipline and denial.

Further, drugs for high blood pressure cause all sorts of unpleasant side-effects. One reason for patient noncompliance is that the patient usually feels quite well before treatment but feels miserable when the drugs are started. This is particularly evident in runners who find that their running capacity is usually cut in half.

Q: I am 44 and recently took a stress test. I found I have a problem with hypertension. I have been seeing a doctor for about six months. My average blood pressure has been 140/100. During the past two months, I've been on medication. It would seem that all the miles I put in over the years have contributed to only a partially sound cardio-vascular system. What is your comment?

A: You are just another victim of the medical establishment. Right now, blood pressure is popular and the medical media are pushing it.

An average blood pressure of 140/100 will still get you standard rating in many insurance companies. And until doctors came under this publication barrage, it would not have warranted treatment.

Too much is made over blood pressure. Frequently, it is only elevated when taken. In World War II, many of the draftees had high blood pressure on examination. In New York, they were sent to Governor's Island where blood pressures were taken periodically. When the blood pressure became normal, they were given a uniform. Most of these "hypertensive" draftees are still around, still getting high blood pressure only when examined.

If anything, running will lower the blood pressure. Several studies have been done to show the beneficial effect of exercise in this area.

I have found the quickest way to find your true normal blood pressure is to hyperventilate. Relaxed overbreathing eliminates any effect of tension. I have seen blood pressures drop by 30 points by this method.

LOW BLOOD PRESSURE

Q: The last time I was examined by a doctor, I was told I had low blood pressure and to watch it. I have been running for more than five years, and yet when I make a long run with friends, it takes me two days to recover. They, on the other hand, are fully recovered the next day. Could this be related to my low blood pressure and, if so, is there anything I can do to improve this condition?

A: Low blood pressure is common in distance runners. It becomes a problem when it is "orthostatic"—a condition where the blood pressure goes down when you stand up.

When this happens, it usually means you are overtrained or in an exhausted state. Your story suggests that you exhaust easily. You are a runner who needs a fair amount of time to snap back and recoup.

Accept that. We are all different. Many people can run only every other day. Some can only run every third day. Each of us is an experiment of one, and no one else's training program can be the same as yours.

I suggest you train on alternate days at a conversational pace and take an hour nap each day off. Increase distance and pace, but be sure to take 1-3 days off a week.

BLOOD TESTS

Dr. Nicholas Newton of the Mission Viejo Club used daily white blood cell counts to monitor training of six top swimmers, including world recordholder Shirley Babashoff.

When counts went to 12,000-15,000, swimmers altered their training pattern, either by skipping practice or easing off, usually to one-third or two-thirds of the workload.

It has been reported that the East Germans have used other data for similar purposes. Tests include blood lactate, urea, creatine phosphokinase and hemoglobin.

Dr. Lloyd Drake of New Zealand, who has advised Olympic 1500-meter champion John Walker, recommends doing hemoglobin tests every two weeks. If he finds the level falling, then they are done every week. A fall in hemoglobin seems to coincide with staleness, poor performance and stress injuries.

However, Brotherhood in England has shown this low hemoglobin is not due to a drop in hemoglobin but a rise in blood volume. Trained athletes develop an anemia which is more apparent than real. According to D. B. Dill and his co-workers at the Desert Research Center in Nevada, the champion athlete has "thin" blood. But he has so much of it his total hemoglobin exceeds that of non-athletes.

HEMOGLOBIN LEVELS

Q: In Fred Wilt's book, *Run, Run, Run*, he reports that Finnish coach Kalevi Rompotti feels that a runner in condition should have 15-16 grams of hemoglobin per 100 cubic centimeters of blood, and at least 4.7 million red corpuscles per cubic millimeter. He says if these values are only 13-14 and 4.2-4.5, one should train with caution. If they are 12.5 and 4.0, he should rest and take medication.

I was recently checked by my physician and received readings of 14.5 grams of hemoglobin and 4.0-4.5 million (estimated) red corpuscles per cubic millimeter. I expressed a little concern that my readings did not reach the levels advocated by Rompotti. But my doctor (not only a capable internist but also a runner) felt that the coach's standards were not only unrealistic but could possibly border on the dangerous. Who's right and why?

A: Both your doctor and Rompotti are right. High hemoglobins have been used to indicate good condition. However, my recollection is that such levels occur only in sprinters and quarter-milers. D. B. Dill reported at the American College of Sports Medicine that a distance runner's hemoglobin actually falls as his condition improves.

This is not a true anemia. The runner's actual hemoglobin increases, but because of a greater increase of plasma volume, the concentration of hemoglobin falls.

So your levels (which are within normal range) would indicate you are in good condition. Should they fall to those cautionary levels mentioned by Rompotti, they could mean you were overtrained.

One Canadian researcher has already used low hemoglobins (a drop of two grams) to indicate overtraining. If he is correct, rest would restore the blood to normal levels. No therapy would be needed. This could be a relatively simple way to follow a runner's progress.

The most interesting "anemia" due to training occurs in horses. Under a program of frequent stressful competition and speed training, a horse's hemoglobin may fall as low as nine grams. Many trainers use the hemoglobin as a guide for training or withholding training and also as an indication of when the horse is ready for a good race.

FAT LEVELS

Q: I've been running 30 miles a week for the past three years, but the cholesterol level on my annual physical has shown little change. How can that be? Shouldn't that amount of running lower my cholesterol?

A: The experts who made such a big thing about cholesterol are now telling us that there is "good cholesterol" and "bad cholesterol." In other words, the absolute level of cholesterol should not concern us too much. What is important is the level of the good cholesterol, the high-density lipids. When they are elevated, you have less likelihood of having coronary heart disease. Running elevates the level of the high-density lipids. This has been demonstrated by Dr. Peter Wood at Stanford who has studied a number of non-runners and runners, and correlated their cholesterol, high-density and low-density lipids levels. What he discovered was that the highest HDL values occurred in women runners. Next highest was in men runners and sedentary women. The only other factor besides running and being a woman that altered the HDL level favorably was alcohol intake.

The beneficial effect of alcohol on high-density lipids and the coronary risk factors, has been supported not only by Wood's studies (about 30% of his veteran runners took three drinks or more a day) but also by studies of Japanese in California. Those who had the least incidence of coronary disease took two beers a day.

How HDL protects against coronary disease is not known. It is theorized that they have a detergent action which prevents or reverses the atherosclerotic processes in the arteries. The important thing to know is that this beneficial effect of running on HDL will not be reflected in the total cholesterol level. That level may remain unchanged while you are actually lowering your risk factors for coronary artery disease. That seems to be happening in your case. Have your doctor test your HDL level.

Q: Is it dangerous to run with a high triglycerides reading? Mine is 227, and my cholesterol level is 136. My doctor said I could exercise but to cut down on my sugar intake. I have been running for four years and now do five miles five times a week. My weight is 170 pounds, height 5'8", age 50.

A: I agree with your doctor. You have a Type IV hyperlipi-demia, the most common type of blood fat disorder. Your cholesterol is quite low, probably as a result of your running program. The high triglycerides are thought, as your doctor said, to be due to excess sugar intake and excess body weight. The recommended diet is one in which carbohydrates are limited to 40% of the daily calories. Alcohol should be restricted and probably avoided.

From your statistics, it does seem as if you can lose some weight. You should use your weight at about age 20 as your standard. It is unlikely that any increase since then has been due to muscle. You now have the incentive to get back to that lean weight. You will probably find that you will run better as you are in the process of reducing your triglycerides.

Q: There is an alternative explanation for the runner with elevated triglycerides. I am a pathologist. Recently, I fasted for 12 hours, ran seven miles and then conducted numerous blood tests. To my surprise and consternation, my triglycerides were elevated. They had always been normal in the past.

I fasted the next evening and re-did the tests the next day without running. The tests were normal. Since then, I've learned that triglycerides are typically elevated after running. This is another hazard runners may face when they have routine physical exams.

A: Generally speaking, we should make it a rule to recheck any abnormal test after a period of inactivity. However, few runners, including myself, are going to give up a day or more of running just to make their physicians feel better. Again, as you say, the normal "abnormality" rears its head and provides another hazard.

BLOOD DONATION

Q: I would like to make an all-out effort to improve my competitive abilities. If I adopt this training program, should I discontinue my current practice of donating a pint of blood to the Red Cross every 60 days?

A: I hate to deprive the Red Cross of those six pints a year, but if you are going into serious training, you had best forget about donating blood.

There is general agreement among physiologists that after blood loss, there is a deterioration of physical performance. Bjorn Ekblom has charted the effect of taking 800 cubic centimeters of blood from three volunteer runners. He found that physical performance capacity decreased by approximately 30%, and maximal oxygen update decreased 13%. The major effects were felt the second day. After that, things began to improve. It took two weeks for the maximum oxygen capacity to return to normal. Heart rate and time for a maximal standard run took four weeks to come to pre-blood-letting standards. The effect of withdrawal of a pint (500 cc.) would be less but still significant.

Anecdotal evidence, mainly from Yale Coach Bob Giegengack, also suggests that competitive runners should forego donating blood. The runner who gives blood runs as if he has mononucleosis, Giegengack told me. He looks okay until the last fourth of the race. When he reaches for his reserve, his acceleration, he finds there is nothing there. Less than maximal effort, however, can be handled without too much difficulty.

NO GUARANTEES

Q: I have a 58-year-old friend who is a race walker. He walks 10-15 miles per day and has completed several 100-mile walks. He also bicycles. Yet, recently, after suffering chest pains, this man was discovered to have coronary heart disease. His cholesterol is in the 250 range. His triglycerides were 244. He's a nonsmoker and about 15% overweight for his height. How do you explain his diseased condition?

A: Your friend in his late 50s is proof that fitness has to do with physiology, not disease. Up until the onset of symptoms, he was performing at the maximum level for his age. Yet all the while, coronary disease was developing in his heart vessels.

His walking and cycling were certainly not wasted. They were enjoyable, allowed him to live each day to the fullest, made him healthy in the complete sense of the word. What they didn't do is protect him from coronary disease. I suspect that he was born with a susceptibility to his disease (his cholesterol and triglycerides are quite high for someone of his weight and physical activity).

This is not to say that walking and cycling may not have a positive effect in retarding the disease or, should an attack occur, in giving a greater chance of recovery. But we shouldn't rely on it. Fitness programs should be evaluated on their immediate effects on our performance, energy, creativity and will power. Longevity, an unproven benefit, should be looked upon as a bonus.

UNTRUE TEST

Q: My doctor has advised me to quit running as a result of two blood tests he has taken. I'm sending you the results. My cardiogram proved normal. I have been running 16 years and racing the last 19 months. I do about 40-50 miles a week. I haven't stopped running yet, but I am puzzled.

A: Don't worry about your tests. They are within the range seen in runners doing your mileage. They do not represent anything serious going on in your body. Our best guess is that these abnormalities occur due to a rapid turnover in muscle metabolism. There is a continual, relatively massive breakdown and buildup of muscle tissue.

The usual annual physical done by physicians leans heavily on laboratory tests. These frequently create hazards for a runner in heavy training. I once received a letter from a 50-year-old daily runner whose tests showed, his physician said, that he had "the liver and kidneys of a 70-year-old alcoholic." What he had, of course, was the usual elevations of blood urea, and the muscle and liver enzymes seen in high mileage runners.

Dr. Joan Ullyot once said she was able to tell from a premarathon profile those who would do badly—the ones with perfectly normal blood counts and blood profiles. Well-trained runners are likely to show low hematocrits along with elevations of various enzymes. I test myself infrequently but always know that when the readings are normal I haven't been training enough.

The advice given by your doctor is the conventional wisdom of the spectator watching someone do some unimportant, nonsensical thing. Admonitions to stop running should not be given without a working knowledge of the normal effects of running on the body.

PART SIX:
RESPIRATORY SYSTEM

*"Faulty breathing is almost universal.
Most of us breathe 'backward.'"*

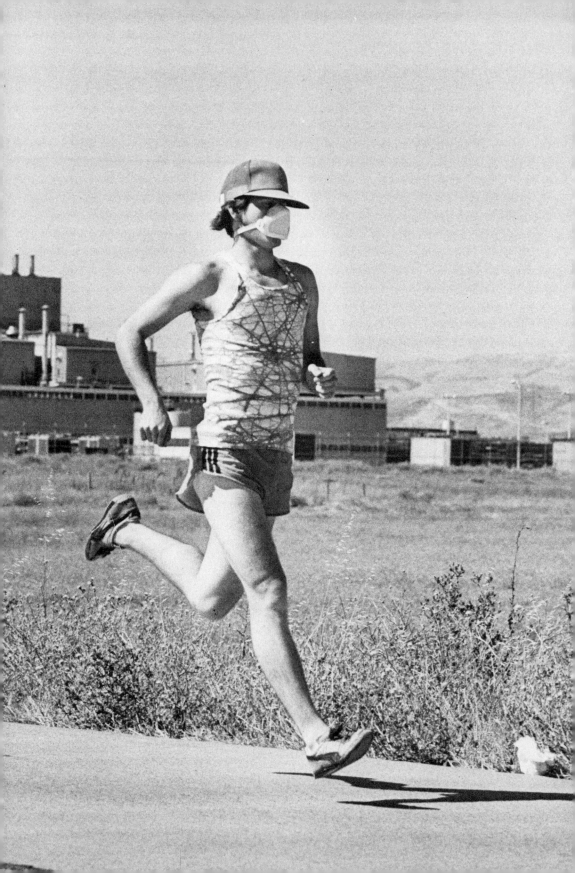

Chapter 24
Clearing the Air

The healthy human body works in silence, and we are unaware of its marvelous workings when things go well. The respiratory tract is no exception. We arise in the morning not even thinking about breathing 16 times a minute for the rest of the day.

However, abnormal function or illness of the respiratory tract can be annoying and even disabling to the runner. And as is usual in most of our overuse syndromes, a predisposition to these disorders and errors in our techniques cause them. Allergies and faulty breathing are the main culprits here.

The allergies are usually indicated by past history of food allergy, hay fever, frequent sneezing, hives, etc. Having a constantly runny nose or being addicted to an over-the-counter nasal spray is also evidence of an allergic problem.

Allergies promote a chronic broncho-sinusitis condition as well as exercise-induced asthma and asthma itself. The ubiquitous "stitch"—a sharp pain in the side—also may well have an allergic component.

The role of pollutants in chronic allergic responses and allergic diseases is less clear. It could be that most pollutants are clinically significant only in the runner with a respiratory allergic condition.

Of course, in every allergic condition the homeostatis of the body is of great importance. Therefore, stress, exhaustion and overtraining can precipitate or prolong any allergic disease.

Faulty breathing is almost universal. Most of us breathe "backward." Instead of pulling in air with our belly, we pull it in with our chest. When we breathe in, our bellies should go out. If, however, I had you stand up and take a deep breath, your belly probably would go in.

Correct breathing is "belly breathing." With belly breathing, the diaphragm moves up and down like a piston, the way it should. With chest breathing, it goes sideways, is ineffective and can go into spasm like a charley horse of the thigh, thus giving the stitch.

In addition to belly breathing, attention must be given to breathing out against pressure. This keeps the tiny bronchial tubes open and prevents "air trapping." Otherwise, it is possible to have a liter of air contributing to distention of the chest and production of the stitch.

The best way to prevent air trapping is by groaning or grunting on exhalation. Bill Bowerman, the 1972 Olympic coach, had his runners breathe out against pursed lips.

Belly breathing is done naturally only when we are on all fours. While standing, it is a willed act. First, it must be learned. Lie on your back on the floor. Put a book on your belly. Then breathe in and out, making the belly rise with inhalation, fall with exhalation.

Then, translate this to running. Fill your belly with air first, then the chest. Push the air out with your belly, and groan to your heart's content.

Whether the runner has a respiratory problem or not, belly breathing is the best way to get oxygen into the body and carbon dioxide out.

Chapter 25
Bad Breathing

OUT OF BREATH

Q: I have been running less than a year and have gotten stuck in the two-mile range for several months. The only impediment to increasing my mileage is either faulty breathing technique or poor lung capacity. By the end of my run, I am panting so hard I sound like a train. All other systems seem to be "go." What suggestions can you make?

A: Incorrect pace rather than incorrect breathing is usually the problem in the inability to extend mileage. You should run at a pace at which you can converse with a companion (the "talk test"). You should also run quite slowly until you begin to perspire. This will occur at about 6-10 minutes. At that point, you will find you can increase speed without increasing effort.

It is true that most runners breath incorrectly. You should learn to belly breathe and to give an occasional foghorn groan to clear your lungs of trapped air. But in the final analysis, pace is the critical factor.

"DR. BREATH"

Q: Is there any system of breathing training designed to strengthen and increase breathing efficiency currently used by runners?

A: Carl Stough (author of *Dr. Breath*) impressed both

coaches and athletes in the pre-Olympic camp at South Lake Tahoe in 1968. Unfortunately, there has been no follow-up on that. I have written to Stough but have never gotten any further indication of his interest.

Percy Cerutty, the unorthodox coach from Australia, was another who claimed that most runners breathe incorrectly. He suggested that we raise our arms away from the body as we inhale.

I would opt for a good singing teacher. It is the combined use of the abdominal and chest breathing used by concert singers that maximizes air intake. Also, expelling air against pressure as singers do causes optimal exhalation of air.

I usually suggest training in abdominal breathing plus exhalation through pursed lips. Breathing should then be synchronized with your pace, exhaling every fourth or sixth step. The aim is to breathe with maximum effect and minimum effort. Studies have shown that respiratory efforts become increasingly inefficient as runners begin to tire.

Q: You mention *Dr. Breath* by Carl Stough. Where and how might I obtain a copy for my own library?

A: *Dr. Breath* can be obtained from the Stough Institute, 54 West 16th Street, New York, NY 10011.

NOSE BREATHING

Q: I am 54 years old and run six miles a day, averaging about eight minutes a mile. For the past two months, I've been experimenting with breathing exclusively through my nose to try to equip myself better for winter running. Am I being stupid? Are there any long-range ill effects to the sinuses or cardiovascular system that can occur from doing this?

A: The nasal passage are not adequate for the air intake necessary in vigorous running. It makes no sense, furthermore, to take air in that way. What you need is to fill the lungs adequately and as rapidly as possible.

The one possible reason I can think of for inspiring through the nose would be to heat the air. However, we know from Carl Gisolfi's experiments in Iowa that this is unnecessary. He proved that air was heated well by the time it reached the bronchial tubes, even in open-mouth breathing.

Discharging air through the nose makes more sense. It provides a resistance which keeps the smaller bronchial tubes open. This situation usually is maintained by pursed-lip breathing or grunting.

EXTRA OXYGEN

Q: I have noted that tennis and football players have resorted to the administration of oxygen during their matches. I would appreciate it if you would give me information on the subject as it might apply to runners.

A: I am willing to be enlightened on this, but I doubt if supplemental oxygen is necessary for athletes except under emergency conditions. The Japanese swimmers introduced oxygen to the sports world as an aid to performance, but I don't see this equipment in use anymore. And this is a time when a world swimming record may last only between a heat and a final.

SIDE STITCHES

Q: For over a year, I've been bothered by pains in my right side whenever I run. I have tried everything—running it off, laying off of running, etc. But whenever I go back to a certain distance and pace, the problem returns. What is it and what can be done?

A: Although you do not give the exact location of your pain, I assume that the discomfort is in the upper abdomen or lower chest, an area which usually is the site of the runner's stitch. This may result from specific muscle weaknesses. I have been struck by the frequency of such weaknesses in runners' abdominal muscles.

Try this yourself. Lie on your back, hands clasped behind your head, knees bent and feet on the floor. Then, try to sit up. If you have difficulty, you have a weakness that needs correcting.

In addition to muscle exercises, I suggest that you work on abdominal breathing with stretching of your belly muscles.

Belly breathing is the most efficient way to breathe. The first exercise for this is to lie on your back on the floor. Then, place your hand or a book on your stomach. It should rise as you breathe in, descend as you exhale.

One other tip that may help is to raise your arms up and out as you inhale while running, and then drop them as you exhale. Moving the elbows forward and backward restricts the air intake to the lungs.

Q: The other day, I got a sideache and found that as I altered my breathing to deep abdomen breathing rather than chest, the pain disappeared almost immediately. I'm sure that correct breathing can have enormous effects on endurance and speed.

A: You have discovered on one run what it took me years to figure out: belly breathing plus exhaling against resistance is the answer to the stitch. It is also the formula for correct breathing.

Another maneuver recommended by running doctor David Worthen is to increase your breathing rate so that it is double your normal rate. He has found this quite effective during a run.

Q: Occasionally, I get cramps in the right side of my upper abdomen which sometimes move into my right shoulder. As I have recently been found to have a floating kidney, my doctor feels the cramps may be caused by the kidney moving up into this region. He has suggested I use a brace while running. The brace chafes, is uncomfortable and does not relieve the cramping pains.

Does the floating kidney cause the cramping pains? Is this anomaly caused by running? Can you tell me how to alleviate the pains?

A: It seems to me that your pain is not related to your kidney at all. The pain appears to be the familiar and controversial stitch.

My experience with this is that it is no less than a charley horse or cramp of the diaphragm. The pain in the shoulder confirms this or is consistent with it.

I would dispense with the brace, learn to breathe correctly with your diaphragm and to breathe out against resistance.

Chapter 26
Respiratory Problems

COMPLICATIONS

Many respiratory complications can interfere with the free flow of a runner's air. I'll detail the key ones:

• *Sinusitis.* Persistent nasal stuffiness, discharge and night cough occur frequently in runners, often as an aftermath of a cold. Any cold, for instance, that lasts more than 10 days must be assumed to have become sinusitis. The nose may be clear, and only by examination will the sinuses be found filled with infection.

Antibiotics are useless in such a condition. Only by expelling this material through douching or lavage will the sinuses clear. Occasionally, self-medication with a nasal spray morning and night, followed by a nasal douche, will help.

Some persistent sinusitis is allergic. Symptoms are much the same, but inspection of the nose tells the story. With infection, the internal nasal structures are red and angry. In allergic situations, they are pale and boggy.

In both types of sinusitis, exhaustion and overtraining may well contribute. The common cold and activation of allergies are two of the most common manifestations of overuse of the body.

Treatment: (1) Over-the-counter nasal spray; at times may have to go to second nasal spray or even, in severe allergy, short course of steroids; (2) drainage of sinuses by physician in resistant infectious cases; (3) humidification of house; optimum humidity is 35%; at least sleeping quarters should be taken care of; (4) reduction of allergies; (5) oral medications, antihistamines and decongestants; however, these have some side-effects and should be avoided if possible; (6) reduce training program.

• *Bronchitis.* It rarely exists alone. The correct term should be broncho-sinusitis. The two areas are in constant communication. Usually, when the bronchial tubes are involved the cough becomes productive, while in sinusitis alone it is mostly dry and nocturnal.

At times, there is an allergic component and asthmatic bronchitis ensues.

Treatment: (1) Do all indicated procedures for sinusitis which probably coexists; (2) steam inhalation (use kettle on stove morning and bedtime); (3) expectorant cough mixture (over-the-counter); (4) antibiotics, if sputum is at all colored and not white; (5) use therapy for asthma if asthmatic bronchitis is present.

• *Asthma.* Asthma, either spontaneous or exercise-induced, is one of the most disturbing problems a runner can have. However, my experience is that most victims of these diseases can be helped, and almost all can learn to run comfortably.

First, we must realize that asthmatic swimmers do extremely well and asthmatic cyclists almost as well. The difference, it seems to me, is that swimmers belly breathe and exhale against pressure. The leaning forward of the cyclist automatically promotes belly breathing.

Asthmatic symptoms may occur during or immediately after running.

Treatment: (1) Correct breathing techniques; (2) previous therapies used for allergic broncho-sinusitis; (3) if this fails, escalate therapy through: Slophylin or Brondelon by mouth. Super inhalations or Bronkometer prior to running. Chromolyn inhalations, Vanceril, a steroid inhalant. All of these, of course, must be under the direction of a physician.

• *Viral pneumonia, pleurisy, etc.* Infections involving the respiratory tract are usually self-limited. The runner's problem is when to return to running.

A study was done by Goran Friman on "The Effect of Infectious Disease on Circulatory Function" which tries to answer this. This study showed that at 3½ months after the illness ended, male patients attained 79% of their normal level; female patients 72%. It was interesting that well patients given the same amount of bed rest and inactivity showed 90% of capacity.

Also, there was still evidence of a poor reaction to standing. An increase in pulse and drop in blood pressure of significant degree was noted on an eight-minute standing test.

Complete recovery from infectious illness requiring bed rest can, therefore, take longer than 3½ months. The runner will usually be asymptomatic at ordinary activity, however. Only performance and maximum work capacity will be altered.

SINUSITIS

Q: What do you do about sinus problems? I have been a track runner for 12 years and am always in good shape. Whenever I start doing fast, quality workouts, though, I start getting sinusitis. What is best for my condition, and what adjustments in my training do you think I should make?

A: Your recurrent sinusitis is an indication that you are continually overtraining. When you overstress yourself, you break down. In effect, you blow a fuse.

The answer, then, is to recognize this tendency. Change your program to every-other-day hard training, and allow for some time off. I recommend recording the basal (first-thing-in-the-morning) pulse and using any significant increase (10 beats) as an indication to slack off.

SORE THROAT

Q: My problem is a chronic sore-throat condition, especially in the colder months. I don't know if work conditions (working all year in a drafty, air-conditioned room), walking (to and from work, about two miles each day) or running (3½ miles a day) causes it.

A: A chronic sore throat is usually due to an allergy or to a persistent sinus infection. Your exercise program may contribute by pushing you into an exhaustion state. This lowers your

ability to handle allergies and reduces your defenses against infections.

A nose and throat specialist, through inspection of your nasal
tissues and your throat, should be able to tell whether you have
an allergy or an infection.

Clearing of the sinuses by Proetz treatments could set you
right. Allergies are, of course, at times matters that would
baffle Sherlock Holmes.

RUNNY NOSE

Q: Do you have any advice for a complaint of constant runny
noses during running sessions outside?

A: The runner's runny nose always seemed to me to be a
blessing. Running and that runny nose act to clear my sinuses
and nasal passages. Whether effort itself is a factor or simply
the irritation of that forced flow of air through the passages
which creates this secretion, I'm not sure.

I see no reason to get into medication for this. The side-
effects could be worse than any help you would get.

SNEEZING

Q: I have been running year round for almost two years and
developed a condition this past winter, sneezing, which has the
doctors baffled. Last March, I started having severe sneezing
spells and a runny nose within 15 minutes of finishing my running. The sneezing and runny nose lasted 4-24 hours. The condition disappeared during the summer and early fall but
returned during a week of running in 50-degree temperatures.
What is your suggestion?

A: These sneezing episodes and runny nose seem to relate to
the following variables: exertion, cold or some local condition in
the nose, and possibly an ingested allergen such as milk, eggs,
citrus fruit, chocolate, etc.

Your cold allergy can be modified to some degree by the time
of day you run. Also, you can wear a ski mask or surgical mask
both to filter the air and warm it up.

If this fails, you might try a prescription nasal spray which
has a steroid, but this seems like overkill to me.

Finally, you might try eliminating the more notorious allergens from your diet.

POST-RUN COUGH

Q: I'm 43 and have been running about five years with mediocre results in competition. Last summer, in an effort to improve my mile time, I started running intervals of 440 in 72 seconds. I immediately developed a severe cough which persisted all summer as I continued the intervals. I stopped them in the fall, and my cough went away. My question is, if I go back to intervals, will my respiratory system adapt, or am I asking for permanent trouble?

A: Post-race cough is a fact of many runners' lives. I know that any all-out race, usually 880 or mile and especially indoors, will leave me coughing for a day or two. I suspect this is due to a drying, irritating effect on the larynx and bronchial tubes. Usually, interval work done at race pace for much shorter intervals doesn't do this.

In your instance, it would seem that either the distance or speed, or both, is too much. I would cut down to 220s or 300s at the same or slower pace. In addition, I would adopt Italian physiologist Rodolfo Margaria's suggestion for speed work: interval 80-100 meters. Theoretically, these can be done indefinitely without building up lactic acid. I have done 20-25 at one session. This would give you speed and strength to add to your endurance.

PLEURISY

Q: I recently contracted pleurisy in one lung, a result of running in the persistently cold weather of this winter. Will my pleurisy be a recurring problem? Should I abstain from training in frigid weather? Will there be any measurable handicap on my capacity for long-distance training?

A: Pleurisy is a wastebasket diagnosis which includes a number of conditions. Because it is not really specific, it is difficult to say what the course will be.

I will assume, however, that you had some sort of viral pneumonia with pleurisy. If so, it will probaby take several months to recover fully.

Subsequently, you should have no worries about recurrence. However, there may be some permanent adhesions at the site. These can give pain with change in weather conditions, exhaustion and other stresses. In this, they are much like a previously-injured joint or trick knee that signals a change in the internal or external environment. This does not indicate any new or acute problem.

ASTHMA ATTACKS

Q: I'm an asthmatic female runner, 31 years old, who's been running 4-10 miles almost daily for 7-8 years. I have a problem running in winter weather. After the first 10 minutes, I get asthma on the run and have to jog the rest of the way with greatly reduced breathing capacity. How do you handle this problem and asthmatics in general?

A: Exercise-induced asthma may be due to a constellation of causes. First, of course, is the susceptibility. After that come a number of factors:

1. *Allergens.* These can be food or inhalants. Sufferers may need to be desensitized against pollens and molds. They may also have to avoid specific foods, including shellfish, strawberries, eggs, milk.

2. *Pollutants.* It is likely that serious air pollution like ozone and possibly sulfur may precipitate attacks.

3. *Cold.* We know that exercise asthma can be worsened in cold weather. Oddly, this is apparently due to the cold air on the face, not in the bronchial tubes.

4. *Incorrect breathing.* Chest breathing instead of correct diaphragm breathing seems to worsen the asthma.

5. *Small bronchial tube collapse.* Due to the allergy or pollutants, small vessels collapse, trapping air and increasing symptoms.

Intelligent therapy should begin with treating these factors before going to drugs. Use of a ski mask, belly breathing and exhalation against resistance may give relief.

HAY FEVER

Q: I have hay fever and take medication to combat it.

Should I stop runing during this time, which is usually about four weeks, or would it be possible to continue with my running? Although I normally run about 10 miles a day, last year I ran only two a day during the hay fever season.

A: I see no need to stop running because of hay fever. If the medication is effective and doesn't decrease your energy level, stay with it.

You might want to try a nasal spray as a substitute or adjunct. There are at least six drug categories or antihistamines. You should be able to find one that is effective and won't interfere with your running.

SMOKING

Q: Please help! What is the effect of smoking on running? At 35 years of age with five years of marathoning experience, the old devil cigarettes returned.

A: Smoking reduces your maximum oxygen capacity and, therefore, your peak endurance efforts. However, this may not be enough of an incentive for you to quit. I would, in fact, be surprised if it were.

Returning to smoking suggests psychological factors operating which are not being overcome by your distance running. Possibly, too, you are overtraining into a depression.

Smoking is a symptom, and resumption of smoking means you should evaluate your lifestyle to see where the problem is.

Q: My problem is smoking. I was smoking two packs a day when I decided to start running. Though I am now in good enough condition to race, I can't stop smoking. I still smoke about 12-15 cigarettes daily. I actually quit for eight days once, but my wife said I became unbearable.

A: I do not believe that, of itself, smoking cigarettes is quite as destructive as the medical profession claims.

I would advise you to accept your present level of smoking. You are obviously a new man since you resumed running, but I doubt that the running can contribute much more to the psychological and physiological needs the 15 cigarettes supply.

True, there are methods to use: hypnosis, transcendental

meditation, "smoke-enders." But you may substitute some other habit or addiction. Further, 15 cigarettes a day has little potential for present or future harm. It does decrease your running performance. But balance that against the person you are when you stop smoking. These changes are real and immediate. Weight gain, irritability and nervous tension seem too great a price to pay to say you have licked smoking.

Smoking at the two-pack level definitely increases your chances of lung cancer. But at your present consumption, neither lung nor cardiac problems become statistically more numerous.

A new look at yourself, a look at where you are and where you are going is what you need. It may not be possible to rid yourself of your problems, but identifying them is an important first step.

PART SEVEN:
GASTROINTESTINAL
SYSTEM

"The staff of life (bread) and the perfect food for young mammals (milk) may be exactly what you can't eat."

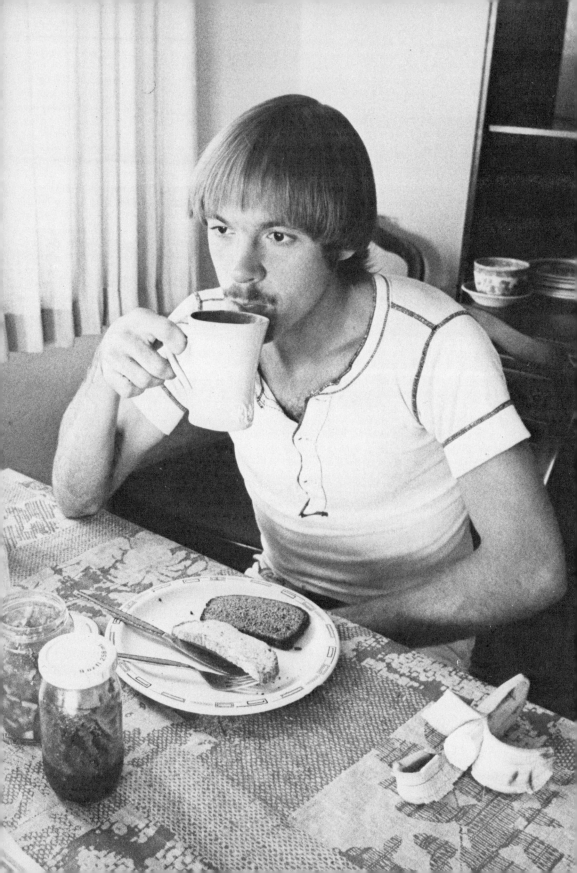

Chapter 27
Few Words on Diet

I gave a talk to a group of runners in New York City. It went well until the discussion period, when the first question was on diet.

I replied, "Well, I don't care much about diet. I don't talk about it."

Then, the fellow asking the question insisted it was advertised that I would say a few words about diet.

I said, "I just have."

I have discovered that people get very subjective and emotional about diet. This is not surprising if you study nutritional anthropology, because there you will find out how much religion has influenced our dietary habits. So I avoid talk about fasting and vegetarianism. And when asked about bee pollen and megavitamins, and trace elements and food supplements, I usually say, "Whatever turns you on."

But there is one demand, an extremely practical one, that I make of a diet: that it doesn't interfere directly with my running.

Unfortunately, as many distance runners can attest, this desired property is at times quite elusive. Many of us apparently have food intolerances of which we remain unaware, mostly because they only surface when we put ourselves under the stress of hard training or competition.

The two main culprits are lactose, which is milk sugar, and gluten, which is found in all grains except corn and rice. Unlikely as it seems, we runners may be done in by bread and milk.

Milk is the major enemy. Despite what centuries of mothers have led us to believe, milk is not the perfect food for young mammals. In fact, almost the entire populations of Asia and Africa have trouble digesting milk. About 6% of white Americans also have this difficulty.

The malabsorption comes in degrees. The amount of milk that will be troublesome varies from one person to another, and this sensitivity apparently is greatly increased by hard running. The end result is gas, distention, noise, discomfort and eventually a large volume of liquid stool that demands to get out.

Likewise, some grain products may cause runners inconvenience, discomfort or embarrassment. This may happen during hard runs and at no other time.

I recommend keeping a food diary, and eliminating items and changing eating times until you find what caused the trouble. Then, limit yourself to the foods and the times you know agree with you.

The only dietary rules I propose are these:

1. Eat foods that agree with you.
2. Avoid foods that disagree with you.
3. Always run on an empty stomach and colon.

The late Dr. Henry Cabot, one of the greatest minds in medicine, once remarked that what would embarrass doctors the most when the Last Trumpet sounded and they heard their Final Judgment would be the diets they had prescribed.

I personally prefer the lean, hungry look and the most palatable diet that will go with it. There are certain minimal daily requirements of protein, carbohydrate, vitamins and minerals which may stand the test of time, although I am not certain. I am certain, however, that we eat too much—too many calories, too much salt, too much sugar, too much distilled liquor. Gandhi said if we are to restrain ourselves and control our lives, we must start with the palate.

Anthropology, which shows us people thriving on very odd diets indeed, should make us as tolerant of another's nutritional behavior as we have become of his economic, social and political activities. There are, it appears, many roads to the promised land. Life, liberty, the pursuit of happiness and a maximum productive lifespan may be found in three visits a day to McDonald's.

The best judge is still your body. How does it look? How does it feel? How does it perform? Find these things out yourself.

Chapter 28
What Runners Eat

PRE-RUN DIET

Q: What are your general recommendations on eating before training and racing?

A: I like a high-protein breakfast with a minimum of carbohydrate. I run about five hours later, usually taking plenty of fluids with some sugar. Then, in the evening, I eat a balanced meal along with sufficient carbohydrate to make up for what I spent in my run. I estimate this at 100 calories per mile. This replaces the sugar in my muscles for my next run.

Most athletes eat a major meal not less than four hours before the event. Some liquids can be taken within 30 minutes. However, if high-sugar drinks are taken 45 minutes to an hour before a long run, hypoglycemia (low blood sugar) may develop during the run.

RUNNING ON EMPTY

Q: I run 3-5 miles about four times a week. I start my run each morning at 5:30, after a five-minute warmup of calisthenics. Is the fact that I run on an empty stomach in any way harmful?

A: Unless it is very hot and humid so that you require extra fluids, it is much better to run without eating. When I run in the morning, if I eat, I have more time to reconsider and some-

198

times go back to bed. Also, I have found that even a light breakfast can provoke a bowel movement midway in the run, which at the very least is an embarrassment.

But perhaps most important, there is no need for any extra calories to take you through the distances you run, and exertion after eating frequently causes disturbances in the circulatory system which can be distressing.

NO APPETITE

Q: Florida heat takes quite a toll in body fluids. I run before dinner. Unfortunately, the quantity of liquid that my thirst demands reduces my appetite and seems to cause improper digestion. Since I am 6'1½'' and 145 pounds, I need to gain weight, not lose it. How do I replenish body liquids without these undesirable side-effects?

A: Running just before dinner reduces appetite whatever the fluid balance problems are. In your instance, the effect is undesirable. But for those of us that have to battle weight, it is an additional reason to run at that time.

It is probable in your case that this ordinary suppression of appetite is enhanced by poor absorption of liquids. Dr. David Costill has demonstrated that half-strength Gatorade, or its equivalent, is absorbed better than the full-strength solution. Reducing the sugar content apparently does the trick.

You can check your total fluid needs by recording your weight before and after the run.

SWEET TOOTH

Q: Since I began running, I find myself craving carbohydrate foods such as ice cream, cookies, fruits, etc., almost to the point that now they are an obsession with me. Is this common with distance runners?

A: I share this attraction with you. I hold myself in check most of the day, but from 8 p.m. to bedtime, I'm an eating maniac. For this reason, despite the extra 700 calories I earn through my hour on the roads, my weight fluctuates a good deal.

Obesity, someone said, begins at 6 p.m. It is easy to control yourself up until then. But then what?

I use fruit, cottage cheese, yogurt and tea, and try to avoid refined sugars. Another device is to eat a saltine with a thick layer of margarine. Fats (preferably saturated) slow stomach-emptying.

ENERGY DRAIN

Q: On a 12-mile run, somewhere between 8½ and 9½ miles I experienced a very sudden energy drain. My legs felt weak, my head was light, and I became extremely thirsty. I walked a short distance and hitched a ride for a mile before I was able to plod home. I have run this distance before with no problem. Did I hit "The Wall"?

A: There are many good reasons to be running, suddenly get this "all gone" feeling and be reduced to a walk. More often than not, this occurs in a race and usually in unseasonably hot weather. I recall walking at the nine-mile mark in a half-marathon on a hot April day.

However, it also can occur if a large amount of sugar is taken about 45-60 minutes prior to running. This sets the stage for hypoglycemia to occur about 30-40 minutes into the run. Therefore, sugared drinks should be taken in the final 15 minutes before setting out on the road.

Another cause of exhaustion would be glycogen depletion of the muscles. This occurs with fasting or in the depletion phase of carbohydrate loading. There are also people who may take several days to replace glycogen depleted by an ordinary training run. Hence, some runners lean toward every-other-day or even every-third-day training.

LOW BLOOD SUGAR

Q: Approximately one year ago, I started a vigorous exercise program that included running two miles per day. With the onset of low blood sugar problems, this exercise program has been curtailed. My usual symptoms are fatigue around meal time and frequent drowsiness when driving an automobile mid-morning or mid-afternoon. I awake in the morning feeling fatigued. I would appreciate your comments.

A: The best remedy for low blood sugar is exercise. The 10 a.m. recess period in school is a good example. At that point, the calories ingested at breakfast have been deposited in the tissues, and the blood sugar is getting low.

The perfect answer is 15 minutes of unrestricted activity. This stimulates the mobilization of sugar from the muscles and builds up the blood sugar. High-protein diet is helpful, as is abstention from coffee and other caffeine beverages. But fitness is the real answer.

I suggest you get back on your running program or some other sport that is really play for you.

Q: I run two miles per day, five days per week. I am also hypoglycemic and am on a prescribed diet. Before running, I have been drinking a glass of orange juice and eating a hard boiled egg, but this does not hold me. What can you suggest for hypoglycemics who want to run or do any prolonged activity?

A: The object in treating hypoglycemia is to avoid stimulating the hyperactive insulin response. So follow a high-protein diet and use complex carbohydrates. Simple sugars must be avoided because they are quickly absorbed, give a quick rise in the blood sugar, and a rapid outpouring of insulin results. In a short time, the blood sugar is driven down to a point where you have symptoms.

The runner must get sugar somehow, yet avoid the hypoglycemia. How to do this?

Recent research suggests what can be done. First, take your high-protein, high-fat meal two or three hours before the run. Then, a minute or so before you run, drink the orange juice. The exercise will slow down the blood sugar rise and avoid the excess insulin response. After that, sugar drinks should be taken every 30 minutes during the exercise.

If the juice is taken too early before starting running, the insulin response will go into action too soon. Running or exercising could end in hypoglycemia.

One corollary to all this: no food, no hypoglycemia. Hence, the early-morning run, before breakfast, may be the best routine for those unable to handle it any other way. However, I suspect if you try this juice-at-the-start routine and something every 30 minutes thereafter, you will do well.

CARBOHYDRATE LOADING

Q: I am prone to gain weight, and when I go through the carbohydrate depletion/loading routine the week before a marathon, I gain too much weight. Is this due to the fact that I taper my running during that week, or is it because of the depletion/loading?

A: Almost everyone gains weight when they taper training if they don't also taper their food intake.

My present feeling about carbohydrate loading is in line with Arthur Lydiard's. Do not deplete with three days of high-protein/low-carbohydrate eating. This obviously weakens you, as most people who have done it can attest.

Instead, start by eating your regular diet, and then "load" by adding honey or sugar-type candy (not chocolate) to your diet the three days prior to the race.

This method usually does not result in the diarrhea or gastrointestinal upset that so frequently attends loading. You will, to a degree, avoid weight gain, although marginal gain is inevitable with successful loading. The water stored with the glycogen gives the increase in weight. You shed this quickly as you race.

Q: In my opinion, the carbohydrate-loading technique which increases muscle glycogen is a dangerous practice for athletes. The approach has been used by a marathoner who suffered angina-like pain and electrocardiographic abnormalities.

Physiologists who developed the diet properly point out that with the increased glycogen deposit there is an associated deposit of three times as much water (one gram of glycogen is associated with three grams of water). Athletes should seriously consider the effects on performance of the increased weight.

Athletes using this practice should be informed as well that glycogen can destroy muscle fibers. Since glycogen deposits can destroy muscle fibers, what happens to the athlete who does not utilize all of the muscle glycogen he has stored as a result of the carbohydrate-loading technique? Does this have an effect on muscle physiology? The answer is unknown.

Athletes and physicians interested in athletics must ultimately choose whether competitive athletics represents technology vs. technology or man vs. man. I prefer the latter, where there is no place for carbohydrate-loading techniques.

A: I am aware of the problems you point out. In fact, I know the runner who had the EKG changes. Nevertheless, runners are finding that this diet does work. The extra water weight may be more of a theoretical than a practical problem. Then again, this may even be extra protection in hot-weather races.

A stopwatch is the runner's final arbiter in such instances, and my running friends have bought this diet on the basis of its evidence. Time will tell its advantages and disadvantages.

FAT AS FUEL

Q: Dr. Ernst van Aaken claims that by fasting and limiting one's food intake, you can train your body to switch over to burning fat instead of relying on carbohydrates. He claims this process would enable one to run distances of great lengths, i.e., 300-plus miles. I would be interested to hear what you have to say about this.

A: I think all of us are plunging into areas that are speculative. If fat is that important, why should Frank Shorter have only 2% body fat? If fat isn't important, why is Tom Osler running so well on his "Eskimo diet" with practically no carbohydrates?

Frankly, I don't know the answer. Fat is a very funny food. Probably 20-30% goes right out in the stool. Some German experimenters fed 6000 calories of corn oil a day to test subjects, and they lost weight.

What has been suggested is that fat would be the preferred source of energy when operating at sub-maximal level. If that is what we understand Dr. van Aaken to mean, perhaps we can agree. Van Aaken thinks this can be done by fasting. Osler says it can be done by eating. I doubt that either can prove it.

EXTRA SALT

Q: Some people tell us to use salt tablets, some say avoid them completely. Would you settle this question once and for all?

A: Like all discussions of half-truths, the salt-tablet question will never be settled. Heat syndromes are complicated problems, and the physiology involved is often confusing. For this reason, you usually see less than the whole picture presented.

The best we can do in this matter is to assign priorities: Water first. Without it, you can die. Without any other presumably essential element, the worst you can have is muscle cramps.

Water first, adequate fluid replacement. Next come salt and/or potassium. Which one? Probably salt. The unacclimatized athlete has considerable salt in his sweat but not very much potassium. The acclimatized athlete loses less salt and more potassium, but he also handles heat better and needs electrolytes less.

Salt is simply part of a total prescription for heat, not the whole answer.

POTASSIUM LOSS

Q: I have been given the enclosed article (summarized below) by many of my non-running friends with the comment that they knew I was killing myself. I thought some of my running colleagues might be interested in your comments concerning hypokalemia and distance running.

(The article from the *Fort Wayne Journal-Gazette* tells of research at the University of Nebraska by Dr. Kenneth Rose involving potassium deficiencies. He says, "I was conducting tests on a group of runners and found that their levels of serum potassium, a vital bodily substance, fluctuated as their training progressed. When they started out, the potassium levels were at 5.3 milliliters per 100 milliliters of blood. After a few weeks, they dropped to 4.0; then after four months to 3.7. After the track season ended and the students ended their intensive training, the levels returned to normal. What this told us was that distance runners progressively lose potassium, and that's not good. In fact, it can be dangerous. Low potassium is a condition known as hypokalemia, and it affects the muscular tone, including that of the most important muscle—the heart. Variations in potassium level can disrupt heart function.")

A: The finding of low potassium at the end of a long, strenuous racing season suggests that it is part of the exhaustion,
depletion or staleness syndrome. Why Dr. Rose considers this
level dangerous is beyond me. "Frustrating" would be a better
designation, since performance and enjoyment will have
decreased.

We are constructed to excrete potassium and conserve salt.
When we increase our salt intake, we defeat this mechanism
and interfere with muscular performance. For four years, I was
on a low-salt, high-potassium intake and did quite well compe-
titively. I finally succumbed to the smell of frying bacon (which
is heavily salted), but I still think the previous diet was the best
one for an athlete.

Low potassium levels are of interest only to those who train
intensively and are highly competitive runners. Restriction of
salt intake is as important as a high potassium intake in provid-
ing an optimal milieu for muscular function.

Whether the simple introduction of potassium supplements
will help is conjectural. Dr. Rose seems to think so. However,
experience with staleness and overtraining suggests that much
more complex mechanisms are at work, and that the hypokalemia is only one of many laboratory findings.

We know, for instance, that under severe stress like surgery—
but also from effort, heat or even impending examinations—
that people can go into negative nitrogen balance. This is a
catabolic state with breakdown of protein, and potassium loss
could easily occur. Further, such states are not readily reversed
and certainly not by mere administration of potassium.

SUPPLEMENTS

Q: I am 54 years old and have a heel spur. A friend of mine
has recommended taking bone meal, saying it cleared up his
heel spur when nothing else would help. What are your feelings
about bone meal as a therapy for this condition?

A: I have difficulty understanding how bone meal helps what
appears to be essentially a mechanical problem. My approach
would be to restore structural and postural balance. At 54, you

are likely to have significant limitations in flexibility. You should work on that. Heel spur pain usually indicates a weak, totally failing foot, and you need support for the foot rather than a change of diet.

Q: Are vitamin C supplements beneficial to long-distance runners and, if yes, how many grams per day should be taken?

A: The next holy war may be fought over vitamin C. I have already decided to be non-combatant. If you like the theories about vitamin C, follow them. If you don't, forget them. Just know that there is no conclusive scientific evidence for or against it.

Nutrition, to my mind, occupies an area somewhere between religion and science, and is a confusing amalgam of these great subjects.

Chapter 29
What Runners Drink

Q: Is there a "best" drink to take during hot-weather running?

A: Yes, the best drink is water. If you are well trained and acclimatized, water may well be all you will need. I once asked this same question of a researcher in a Midwest university who was working on a commercial replacement fluid for hot weather training. "If we could market water," he answered, "we would." The primary aim of such a solution is to maintain blood volume. Only water can do that. Anything else that is added has to do with performance, not survival. Unlike the other additives, if you don't get enough water you die.

Q: How much water is enough?

A: The recommended minimum intake is 10 ounces at the start and 10 ounces every 20 minutes. The average individual can absorb up to one ounce a minute. At that rate, you can take about two quarts an hour without difficulty.

You should establish your own needs in your training runs. Weigh before and after runs where you consume a quart an hour. Your weight loss will establish any extra need for fluid. One quart weighs 2.2 pounds.

Q: How do you arrange to get fluids?

A: In the race, there are water stations. I have learned to use them. It is worth coming to a full stop to take the prescribed amount of fluid. If I see a runner ahead pass a water stop, I know I will beat him.

For my training runs, I have pre-arranged pitstops. My first drink is at home, of course, then I use a friend's house, the caddy house on a golf course, a gas station or two, and then there is an obliging bridge tender with some ice water in his refrigerator.

Q: So water is good. Is there any way to make it better?

A: Any number of substances have been added to water in the hope of creating a better replacement solution. Those with the greatest enthusiasts include salt, potassium, sugar, caffeine and alcohol. Some drinks have been compounded specifically to combat heat syndromes. They are called "Ades." They have good and bad features.

Q: What are the advantages and the drawbacks of the "Ades."?

A: The advantages are that they are mainly water, and contain sugar, salt and potassium. The disadvantages are that they have too much sugar (except for Body Punch), too much salt (except for ERG). The best solution to these solutions, it seems to me, is to use them one-half strength. When you come to a water station take one cup of water to each cup of "Ade."

Q: Don't I need sugar during a race?

A: I think you need sugar just before and then at regular intervals from one hour on. The "Ades," however, are a 5% solution which slows the absorption of water. Hence, the half-strength recommendation.

Q: How about salt and potassium. Don't we need extra quantities of them?

A: Except for the first week or 10 days of hot-weather running when the sweat contains excessive salt, no extra salt in needed. Added salt slows water absorption and increases the need for potassium. Further, studies done on eight marathon runners who collapsed in the heat at Boston showed that the blood levels of both salt and potassium were actually increased rather than decreased.

I suspect, however, that potassium should be increased in the diet. One convenient method of doing this is to use one of the salt substitutes. They are very low in salt and high in potassium.

Q: You also mentioned caffeine?

A: Caffeine is said to spare muscle sugar and increase the utilization of fats. Helpful or not, caffeine drinks have always been popular with athletes. Frank Shorter leans toward defizzed cola, the oldtimers were big for tea and honey, skiers traditionally use chocolate, and coffee is another pre-race favorite.

Of these, tea suits me best. It also contains theophyline which improves the coronary circulation and opens up the bronchial tubes. I almost always use tea and honey as my pre-race drink on a cold day. On a hot day, I take water, tea, half-strength "Ade" or beer depending on which is available.

Q: Why beer?

A: Beer is a low-sugar mixture, virtually free of salt, with a modest amount of potassium and an extra energy source in alcohol. These alcohol calories differ in not needing digestion. They are almost immediately absorbed, thereby giving a quick energy supply and leaving a low-sugar solution that permits rapid absorption of water.

Q: I am still confused. Which of these drinks are the "best."?

A: I am reminded of Dr. Joslin's answer to the question, "which insulin is the best insulin?" His reply was, "All insulins are good insulins if you know how to use them."

My personal experience favors a replacement drink at the start that has caffeine and sugar, then I shift to plain water for the next 45 minutes (too much sugar not only slows absorption, it can cause diarrhea), and from there on in I prefer something that provides water and quick energy.

That adds up to tea at the start, water in the middle, and tea and honey, Coke, half-strength "Ade" or beer to get me to the finish. Which one depends on the water stations and the crowd. I drink the drink at hand. At some point, the "best drink" becomes whatever is available.

THE BEST DRINK?

Q: Aside from beer, your apparent favorite, what is the best fluid replacement drink?

A: Everyone has a favorite. Frank Shorter uses defizzed Coke, and the Honolulu Marathon also uses a mixture of 70% Coke and 30% water. Others advocate the commercial preparations such as Body Bunch, ERG or Gatorade, but dilute the Gatorade more than the manufacturers recommend. This reduces the sugar concentration. Dr. David Costill has reported that fluids with more than 2.5% sugar, especially with significant amounts of salt, may simply lie in the stomach.

MIXED DRINKS

Q: I've read a number of articles about the importance of fluid and electrolyte replacement, and have found that ERG (Electrolyte Replacement with Glucose) seems to fill the bill nicely without tasting too terrible or having bad after-effects. I assume that during long races one should drink it whenever possible. The question I have concerns the quantity one should consume during a week's training to keep a good chemical balance. I may lose as much as 3-4 pounds during a 15-20-mile run, which I suppose is mostly fluid. This weight of ERG would be about a half-gallon, which seems a bit much to drink.

A: It is David Costill's contention, supported by his testing, that no one can completely replace his fluid loss during a long run on a hot day. It is simply not absorbed from the stomach and sloshes around in there. The runner's intake is, therefore, limited by distention or even nausea caused by the fluid.

There is apparently no danger of getting too much fluid in your system. However, loss of more than 3% body weight from dehydration may result in moderate to severe heat-stress symptoms. Most physiologists are now recommending 10 ounces of fluid every 20 minutes as a prevention. Taking fluid in similar quantity just before a run has also been advised. The object is to remain as close as possible to your starting weight.

Q: What medical problems, if any, could occur by using Body Punch in gelatin capsules? At the Honolulu Marathon, I filled gelatin capsules with Body Punch and swallowed four or five with a glass of water at each aid station. There were 12 aid stations. The only problem I had after the race was blurred vision for about two minutes as I was standing around and waiting for the awards.

A: I think you received more help from the water than you did from the Body Punch. Your post-race episode was probably a drop in blood pressure, the familiar Buckingham Guard Syndrome from standing at attention. Only in this instance, your exhaustion and post-marathon weakness could have been a factor. Lying down is the cure.

It seems to me that dehydration is now the runner's fault. The stations are there, but people seem to worry about losing time and pass them up. This is stupid, to say the least. The time saved is lost to dehydration later on. It is also dangerous. Heat is the only thing that can kill a healthy athlete.

COLA

Q: I have run 30-50 miles a week for six years. Like most runners, I drink quite a bit of liquid each day. Perhaps the only thing I have in common with Frank Shorter is a passion for Coca-Cola. In fact, I drink about 2-3 quarts of cola per day. Time after time, friends have told me, "That stuff will rot your stomach." Is there any evidence that I am indeed placing my digestive tract in danger? If so, what drinks, other than water, would be safe replacements?

A: Cola is a beverage with very few redeeming features except it is delightful to drink. It has sugar which is usually unnecessary, caffeine which is habit-forming at the least, and it is highly acidic.

I doubt, however, that cola initiates any stomach disorder, although it probably contributes to the discomfort should there be any inflammation present.

I was taking the same amount of cola as you for some years but have switched to diet cola. I had the feeling that I would be better off without all those calories. If you switched to diet cola, you probably could drop 5-6 pounds in a month.

COFFEE AND TEA

Q: I sometimes drink a cup of coffee before training. Am I looking for trouble, and is a person who drinks 3-4 cups?

A: I'm not sure how many runners take coffee before they run. I frequently do, especially before a race. Some physicians advise against it in a long race because there may be a letdown about three hours later.

However, for a dedicated coffee drinker like myself, there seems to be no problem. I see no reason not to drink it unless it results in cramps, diarrhea or in some way decreases your performance in the later stages of runs of two hours or more.

Q: Could you briefly comment on the adverse effects caffeine-type drugs have on athletes, and do you feel that drugs of this nature are really harmful to the natural activity of human physiology?

A: Coffee is an excellent stimulant with many unfortunate side-effects. If you can do without the caffeine in coffee, you are much better off. If you can't, it might be worth trying to switch to tea.

I am in the process of increasing my tea intake and hope thereby to cure myself of the coffee habit. After that, I'll get to a substitute for tea.

Q: I would like to know the longterm effects of drinking tea, especially as compared to drinking coffee. I am an avid tea drinker and am hoping that it is not detrimental to my health.

A: Tea is a superior drink to coffee from a scientific basis. It has caffeine but for some reason doesn't give the jitters people occasionally get from coffee. It also contains theophyline which has a beneficial effect on the heart and circulation.

Further, tea doesn't create the gastric problems seen with coffee even if the coffee is decaffeinated.

I know of no particular limits on tea drinking. I am sure there are people who consume huge amounts each day without any noticeable harmful effects.

BEER

Q: I view with some skepticism the conclusions drawn by those who drink beer before or during a race. From my own experience, it seems that beer drinking has three physiological effects.

First, it seems to dehydrate the body, thereby robbing it of valuable fluids needed during a long race.

Second, it causes an increased need to use the toilet, which could be a great embarrassment during a long race.

Most important, we know that beer is one of the best cures for sobriety known to man. On the basis of that alone, it would seem beer consumption disqualifies the imbibing runner.

Your friend, Dr. Bassler, may find great pleasure in "jogging a six-pack," but if he does that during a marathon, he would not be sober at the finish unless it took him eight hours to run the course.

A: Water loss in running is generally through sweating, not through urine formation. The effective blood flow to the kidneys is greatly diminished. Hence, the diuretic action of alcohol seems to be minimal. What actually robs the body of valuable fluids is sweating. I have a friend who dropped out of a terribly hot Boston Marathon at the 15-mile mark. He had lost 12 pounds. This represents more than five quarts of water, none of it lost through urine.

I also know of people who, despite extremely high fluid intake after the marathon, have not urinated until the next day. So, diuretic or not, you need a higher renal blood flow and some excess water to have any significant urine formation.

Even before going to beer, I drank enough fluids on the way to have to urinate once or twice. In fact, Dr. Noel Nequin in Chicago says that the need to urinate twice during a marathon is the best indication that you have taken enough fluid.

You should also note that tea, another established drink, and Coke, which is used extensively in the Honolulu Marathon, also contain a diuretic caffeine. Now, the exercise physiologists tell us caffeine helps mobilize free fatty acids, a prime fuel in long-distance running.

It is one thing to theorize using available information, quite another to put it to the personal test. Running is a chancy sport, and we should be reluctant to see cause and effect too readily. However I can, at a minimum, attest to the absence of any bad side-effects from drinking beer on the run.

Dick Walsh, 54, of Las Vegas, wrote this letter to me after the 1977 Boston Marathon:

> The beer discussion is very interesting, and I'd like to let you know of my own experience involving beer and marathoning.
>
> Prior to the Boston Marathon, my best effort was 3:27. I had run at least two dozen marathons prior to that race, usually in the 3:40 range. The night before Boston, I consumed at least six beers by midnight, along with a pizza. During the marathon, I drank two beers, at about the nine-mile and at the 17-mile mark. I was as a child while running. I stopped at least four times to hug a child or to chat with a girl, etc. I finished with a great euphoria, suffering no hurts whatsoever, in a time of 3:17.
>
> I am happy to see that you do not summarily close yourself off to possibilities of things from left field helping a fellow's running.

SAVE THAT SALIVA?

Q: In light of the need to conserve and consume fluids during long-distance runs, I would like to know how important it is to swallow saliva?

A: To answer this question, you would first have to measure the amount of saliva generated during a race. I know of no such figure. In fact, the only saliva-saver I remember was the young boy in "National Velvet." My recollection is that he finally dropped his collecting bottle full of spit, and the author never gave us a clue to the amount.

I suspect that the quantity of saliva that we spit out is insignificant and no factor in our fluid loss.

However, there is to my knowledge at least one reason besides conserving fluid for swallowing saliva. A pharmacist-runner has reported to me that it helps relieve heartburn.

Chapter 30
Internal Upsets

RUNNING BRINGS IT OUT

For reasons known and obscure, distance runners suffer from many gastrointestinal complaints. These vary from aggravation of pre-existing disease to recurrent, intractable problems whose true causes remain a mystery.

I have experienced many of these signs and symptoms of malfunction, and am still searching for answers. One answer is, of course, my body build and personality. I am an ectomorphic individual who responds to situations with my gut. My bowels are the sounding board of my emotions. I belch and break wind through the day. I awake from time to time with heartburn, and the shape, size and consistency of my bowel movements are an ever-changing surprise.

In my competitive college days, I mostly threw up after races. Now, I have cramps and diarrhea. I am continually seeking diets and medications that will prevent this from happening.

In general, the effect of exercise on the intestinal tract is immediate rather than long-range. During running, the visceral blood supply is reduced from 25% of the cardiac output to about 3%. There is also an increase in propulsion or peristaltic activity. Such activity also increases with tension or stress. Perhaps anticipation of the race, therefore, contributes to the stomach and intestinal activity.

This is not all bad. The passage of gas is frequently the assurance that I have settled down to best pace. A runner-friend told me once, "A farting horse never tires. The farting man's the man to hire."

Running may increase the likelihood of gastric hypersecretion and duodenal ulcer. But I have seen no proof of this. Many distance runners have "ulcer" constitutions, anyway. Stomach and duodenal problems would be part of their life, running or not running. If anything, running is therapy for the tensions that I perceive as ulcerogenic. When I develop symptoms of such disturbance, I continue my running, and it does not delay my recovery.

It does seem, however, that the stress of long training runs or all-out races can make latent problems come to the surface. Intolerance to certain foods or food allergies may only be present under a heavy load of running stress. Diarrhea from lactase deficiency or gluten intolerance are instances of that.

Some of the more distressing gastrointestinal problems in runners are:

Malabsorption syndromes. Various enzymes necessary to the digestion of sugars may be diminished or absent. The most frequently deficient enzyme is lactase. This is usually confined to non-dairy cultures. Africans and Asiatic peoples are most affected. The usual incidence in the United States is put at 10% of whites and 70% of blacks.

The treatment is to reduce the milk and milk products in the diet. Non-pasteurized yogurt can usually be tolerated.

Gluten sensitivity. Although this is present in low numbers of the population, possibly one in 100, strenuous exercise probably makes latent difficulties symptomatic. In such individuals, the bowel is sensitive to gluten. This is present in all grains except rice and corn. Gluten is ubiquitous and a gluten-free diet is quite difficult to maintain. All baked goods, gravies, cereals, (again excepting corn and rice) and many other foods where gluten is in the filler must be avoided.

Irritable colon. The spastic or irritable colon is a dysrhythmic organ which produces considerable gas and ribbonlike stools. Tension and gassy foods contribute, but the basic disturbance seems to be with the autonomic nervous system and its control of bowel function. It is probably a big factor in the cramps and diarrhea of the distance runner.

The diet should be free of gassy foods and any substances liable to come through undigested: corn, nuts, raisins, etc. Recent studies show that 50% of irritable colon patients may also have lactose deficiency.

TOO MUCH MILK

Q: I am a 60-year-old, and for the past 10 years I have been running cross country 3-5 miles almost daily. During the past two or three years, I developed a "gas" condition which seems to be confined to my lower gastro-intestinal area with little if any pain or discomfort. My doctor feels that I have developed an intolerance for milk. My daily consumption was about one quart liquid plus a large bowl of ice cream before retiring.

In the process of removing milk and ice cream from my diet, I lost 10 pounds during a two-week period. The more I lost, the better I felt running. Accordingly, I almost automatically increased my speed or distance run each day.

My gas situation has improved some, but not completely. Unfortunately, I am now very tense and nervous and feel relaxed only when I'm running. When I am at "rest," my muscles twitch, jump and jerk randomly, and I have a creepy, crawly feeling. This interferes with my sleep and has begun to worry me considerably which, of course, makes matters worse.

A: It seems as if your doctor was right. You do have a milk problem (usually caused by an enzyme deficiency). You also may have an intolerance to grain products, giving you the difficulty that remains.

Your symptoms suggest overtraining, and I suggest you cut down to running every other day, giving your body a chance to recoup. I doubt that you are in any serious difficulty.

Q: Having had considerable education and personal experience in the area of nutrition, I take exception to your advice to the 60-year-old runner who gave up dairy products because he could not digest milk protein. I think his nervousness is because of the calcium deficiency, not overtraining as you suggested.

A: The man's problem was inability to digest milk sugar

(lactose). The prescribed diet is not free of dairy products, but of lactose. Yogurt, buttermilk and cheese are allowed. At 60, a man who runs 5-10 miles daily does run the risk of overtraining, and of developing nervousness and agitation as a result.

INCIDENCE OF LACTOSE MALABSORPTION IN ADULTS

POPULATION/AREA	MALABSORBERS
Denmark	1-2%
Switzerland	6%
Whites, US	6-8%
Whites, Australia	6-20%
United Kingdom	10%
Italy	11%
Europe	15-24%
Finland	18%
Puerto Rico	20-60%
India	24-80%
Blacks, Africa	30-90%
Mexican-Americans, US	55%
Indians, US	65-95%
Blacks, US	70-75%
Eskimos, Greenland	72%
Ashkenazik Jews, US & Israel	80%
Aborigines, Australia	80-90%
China	83-97%
Greeks, Cyprus	88%
Japan	90%
Thailand	97%
Indians, South America	100%

ABDOMINAL CRAMPS

Q: My 14-year-old son is running cross-country in high school. He suffers abdominal cramps after every race. These cramps last longer than eight hours and almost double him over. Is there anything he can do to prevent these?

A: Your son's problem appears to me to be the "irritable bowel syndrome" or spastic colon. Running increases the activity of the bowel and any spasm that may be present.

The severity of his symptoms, however, suggests and additional element, possibly milk or grain intolerance. I suggest he avoid milk products and ice cream, and switch to yogurt as a substitute. With milk, it is the milk sugar that is the cause of the difficulty, and that is predigested in the yogurt.

If this fails, he should try a gluten-free diet. No grains except corn and rice are allowed. This means no baked goods, cereals (except corn and rice), bread, gravy or any meat with a filler added. A complete list may be obtained from any dietary manual.

Q: I am a 27-year-old long-distance runner. After workouts of 8-10 miles, I develop pain in my lower stomach, and it is worse when I lean back and take a deep breath or when I cough. What do you think causes this?

A: You have to know whether this pain is in the muscle or in the abdomen itself (colon spasm, for instance).

The next time you have the pain, lie on your back and then push on your stomach until you find the tender area. Now, keeping the legs straight, raise your heels about six inches off the floor (or ground). This action tightens the muscle and protects the abdominal contents.

Now, push again. If it is still tender, your problem is in the muscular wall. If it is no longer tender, it means the pain is deeper.

If the pain is muscular, try bent-leg situps and back bends (with tightening of your buttocks muscles to prevent back pain). If the pain is intestinal, have a bowel movement before the practice, avoid milk and drink tea instead of coffee.

SLOSHING

Q: My stomach makes sloshing noises when I run, even though I run with an empty stomach. Do you have any ideas about what the cause is and how to avoid it?

A: The sloshing may occur at lower levels than the stomach. Fecal matter is liquid through the caecum to the middle third of the colon.

You may try a high-fiber diet or a bulk laxative like Konsyl or Metamucil. Other steps that might help would be to switch from coffee to tea. Also reduce milk and milk products.

DIARRHEA

Q: I get severe gastric disturbances whenever I run long distances. I ran my first marathon and had to stop three times on account of diarrhea. In the second marathon, I took Kaopectate before the run. It helped somewhat, but I still had to stop twice and felt sick the whole time. In my third marathon, even though I felt fitter than ever, I had to quit midway because of intense gas pains.

A: I'm hearing from more and more runners who get gas pains and diarrhea during long races. Most have attributed it to an irritable colon. My own experience is that the irritable colon is not enough to cause the problem. I have this condition and have had severe diarrhea on only one occasion—when I took a quart of milk and a quart of orange juice for my pre-race meal!

I think you shouldn't deviate significantly from your normal foods the day of the race. Most of us try different pre-race meals instead of sticking to our usual breakfast foods we know don't bother us.

Some people have diarrhea occurring reflexively from high stomach acid. Use of Tums or Rolaids just prior to a race may then be helpful.

DRY HEAVES

Q: My problem is "dry heaves." These attacks usually occur at or after the five-mile point in my runs, after or during an uphill run, and during warm and/or humid weather conditions. These are time-consuming, physically draining and psychologically demoralizing. I perspire rather freely, but consume little or no liquid during my runs. What causes these attacks and how can I prevent them?

A: What causes stimulation of the vomiting center? I don't know. Some byproduct of severe anaerobic stress I would guess.

The five-mile mark might be significant to an exercise physiologist. What metabolite peaks at that point? What necessary blood element decreases? Is the pH of the blood a factor?

As you can see, I don't know. I'm not sure anyone knows. I suggest that you try to maintain your body's balance with adequate fluid, electrolyte and sugar intake. Use of an antispasmodic (like Kolyantyl) and an anti-nauseant (like Dramamine) might help.

Q: Your suggestion to use Dramamine to combat vomiting has almost solved my problem. I've been taking the tablet the past two months, but still feel nauseated and sick to my stomach at about 14 miles. Up to this distance, I'm okay. What should I do?

A: I'm happy the Dramamine helped, but it obviously did not get to the cause. Your cutoff point at 14 miles suggests some metabolic crisis. Suggestions would be similar to those advanced to explain "the wall"—depletion of glycogen, low blood volume and development of acidosis.

Any or all of these might be prevented by a vigorous hydration program with a drink containing sugar. I suggest you begin your run, regardless of weather, with 12 ounces of a half-strength fluid replacement drink or its equivalent (diluted, de-fizzed cola, for instance). Then, take something similar in 10-ounce quantities every 20 minutes.

Such a program should give your body the ability to maintain its internal balance. For some reason, it goes out of balance at that 14-mile mark.

ULCERS

Q: I have a nervous stomach condition which at one time resulted in a duodenal ulcer that healed in two weeks. However, I've often wondered if the physiological results of running (the buildup of lactic acid) can aggravate or do permanent harm to my condition. I've been running more than six years now and feel that, if anything, running is beneficial ro me because of the psychological results.

You've mentioned that it is better to run on an empty stomach. Many times, I find that if I eat a suitable foodstuff 30-60 minutes before a run, I feel much better during the run than if my stomach were empty. Any information you can provide would be greatly appreciated.

A: Running, it seems to me, is more likely to help your stomach than not. Duodenal ulcers are (for reasons we don't know) seasonal. They also seem to be related to psychological stress. Since running seems to relieve stress and enables the runner to cope with his problems, this would appear to be beneficial.

Your finding that you feel better with food in your stomach (it takes 2-4 hours for it to leave your stomach) must be respected. Listen to your body. You might also try some antacid and an antispasmodic (Kolantyl is such a mixture).

My own observation is that nighttime pain is a sign the stomach is about to erupt. I use Daricin at bedtime for 4-5 days and all quiets down for a few months.

I see no reason these simple measures shouldn't allow you to keep running.

WEIGHT CONTROL

Q: I lost 20-25 pounds the first five months after starting to run. Now, I have leveled off at 155 (I am 5'11"). Everyone says I look weak, skinny, arms thin, no chest, etc. I would like not to look bad. What must I do?

A: Be happy with your appearance. If anyone tells me I look good, I know I'm out of shape—usually 5-10 pounds overweight. Runners should have a lean, hungry look, and from your statistics you may not even now be lean and hungry enough.

Q: In 15 months of running, I have brought my weight down from 250 pounds to 185, but I seem unable to lose any more. I am still 20 pounds shy of my goal of 165, which I weighed as a high school wrestler. What can I do?

A: In high school, you were probably not yet fully developed, so your best weight may be higher than that now. Also, wrestlers have very little body fat, usually on the order of 3-8%, which is very difficult to reach again.

Still, your running has paid off and paid off well. You have hit a plateau which you cannot leave without changing your diet. What you should do is lower your intake by 250-500 calories a day. This will give you a weight loss of a half-pound to one pound a week.

Pick out the major offenders—baked goods, beer, ice cream, candy—and reduce or eliminate them. Try eggs and bacon for breakfast rather than toast and cereal and juice. This will give you a good start and allow you to modify your lunch.

CALORIES USED PER MILE OF RUNNING

WEIGHT				PACE PER MILE					
pounds	*5:20*	*6:00*	*6:40*	*7:20*	*8:00*	*8:40*	*9:20*	*10:00*	*10:40*
120	83	83	81	80	79	78	77	76	75
130	90	89	88	87	85	84	83	82	81
140	97	95	94	93	92	91	89	88	87
150	103	102	101	99	98	97	95	94	93
160	110	109	107	106	104	103	101	100	99
170	117	115	113	112	111	109	107	106	105
180	123	121	120	119	117	115	114	112	111
190	130	128	127	125	123	121	120	118	117
200	137	135	133	131	129	128	126	124	123
210	143	141	139	137	136	134	132	130	129
220	150	148	146	144	142	140	138	136	135

Note: expenditure of 3500 calories equals one-pound weight loss.

CALORIES USED PER MINUTE

WEIGHT				PACE PER MILE					
pounds	*5:20*	*6:00*	*6:40*	*7:20*	*8:00*	*8:40*	*9:20*	*10:00*	*10:40*
120	15.6	13.8	12.1	10.9	9.9	9.0	8.3	7.6	7.0
130	16.9	14.8	13.2	11.8	10.7	9.7	8.9	8.2	7.6
140	18.1	15.9	14.1	12.6	11.5	10.5	9.6	8.8	8.1
150	19.4	17.0	15.1	13.5	12.3	11.2	10.2	9.4	8.7
160	20.6	18.1	16.1	14.5	13.0	11.8	10.9	10.0	9.3
170	21.9	19.2	17.0	15.3	13.8	12.7	11.5	10.6	9.8
180	23.1	20.2	18.0	16.2	14.6	13.3	12.2	11.2	10.4
190	24.4	21.3	19.0	17.0	15.4	14.0	12.9	11.8	10.9
200	25.6	22.4	19.9	17.9	16.2	14.8	13.5	12.4	11.5
210	26.9	23.6	20.9	18.7	17.0	15.5	14.1	13.0	12.1
220	28.1	24.7	21.9	19.6	17.8	16.2	14.8	13.6	12.6

IDEAL WEIGHTS (WOMEN)			
Height	Small Frame	Medium Frame	Large Frame
4'10"	92-98	96-107	104-119
4'11"	94-101	98-110	106-122
5'0"	96-104	101-113	109-125
5'1"	99-107	104-116	112-128
5'2"	102-110	107-119	115-131
5'3"	105-113	110-122	118-134
5'4"	108-116	113-126	121-138
5'5"	111-119	116-130	125-142
5'6"	114-123	120-135	129-146
5'7"	118-127	124-139	133-150
5'8"	122-131	128-143	137-154
5'9"	126-135	132-147	141-158
5'10"	130-140	136-151	145-163
5'11"	134-144	140-155	149-168
6'0"	138-148	144-159	153-173

IDEAL WEIGHTS (MEN)			
Height	Small Frame	Medium Frame	Large Frame
5'2"	112-120	118-129	126-141
5'3"	115-123	121-133	129-144
5'4"	118-126	124-136	132-148
5'5"	121-129	127-139	135-152
5'6"	124-133	130-143	138-156
5'7"	128-137	134-147	142-161
5'8"	132-141	138-152	147-166
5'9"	136-145	142-156	151-170
5'10"	140-150	146-160	155-174
5'11"	144-154	150-165	159-179
6'0"	148-158	154-170	164-184
6'1"	152-162	158-175	168-189
6'2"	156-167	162-180	172-194
6'3"	160-171	167-185	178-199
6'4"	164-175	172-190	182-204

Q: I've read a lot of differing views about ideal weight. Every chart I see varies as to what I ought to weigh. Some charts refer to small, medium and large frames, which makes me suspect ideal weight varies for people the same height. How can I tell my ideal weight?

A: My professor of medicine used to say that your ideal weight was your lean body weight. So the lower the per cent body fat, the better off you are. You probably were at your optimum weight when you graduated from school or were married. Even then, you were probably 15% body fat. Take your weight at that age, reduce it another %, and you are near the figure you want as a runner.

PART EIGHT:
OTHER SYSTEMS

"Sweat cleanses from the inside. It comes from places a shower will never reach."

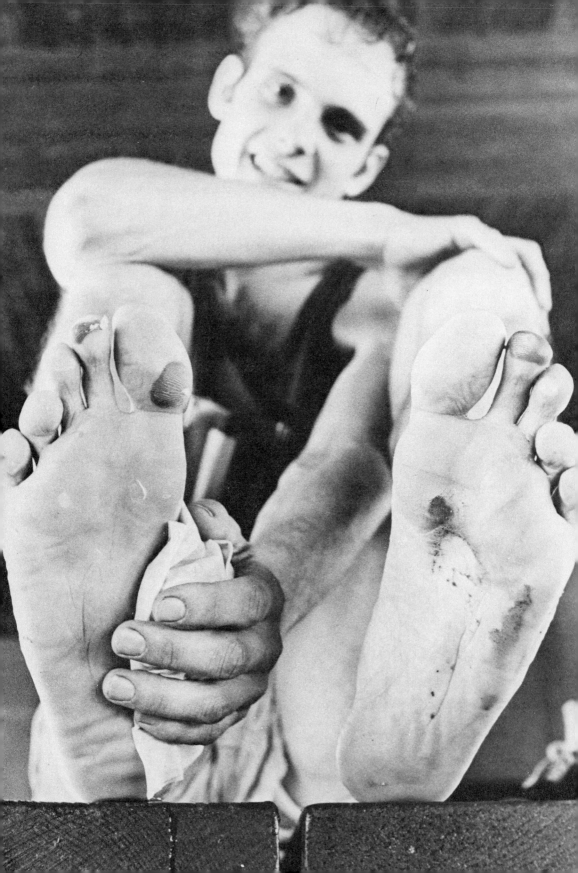

Chapter 31
Skin and Nail Care

BLISTERS

Q: My problem is blisters, especially on the bottom of my right big toe. The best shoes and two pairs of socks don't even seem to help. I hear Dr. Scholl's makes a foam rubber toe cap. Would this help?

A: I suggest you paint or spray the area with tincture of benzoin. Next, tape it with Zonas tape. This is made by Johnson and Johnson and can be obtained in a surgical supply store.

Two pairs of socks won't work. However, the toe cap might be effective. I have had no experience with it, but I have had experience with the benzoin and Zonas tape, and I know they work.

The drawback is that you have to tape for each training session or race. I tend to leave the tape on for days, until it lacerates my skin. Of course, this should be avoided.

Q: I'm prone to blisters. When they develop, what is the best and fastest cure?

A: If the blister is distended with fluid, I may drain it but usually do not take the skin off.

Bandaids or bandages are bad news. They increase the shearing action, and cause more pain and blistering. The usual adhesive tape is too stiff and doesn't follow the contours of the skin, which is why Zonas tape is the best.

ZONAS TAPE

Q: You talked about Zonas tape. I have asked at the drug store and talked with the pharmacist, and no one in our area knows what it is or where it may be purchased.

A: Yours is about the sixth inquiry I have received about Zonas tape. I am inclined to think that pharmacists just don't give a damn. If it isn't on the shelf, the hell with it.

Zonas is a standard product of Johnson and Johnson, the biggest name in the field. It is used routinely by trainers, is found in almost every emergency room and can be obtained in 12-inch rolls (cut to one-inch widths if you so desire) from surgical supply houses.

FOOT TREATMENT

Dr. John Anderson, an Oakland, California veterinarian and runner wrote:

> I would like to expand on your suggestion of putting tincture of benzoin on the toes. Several years ago, Dr. H. C. Smith, a veterinarian in California, published a formula to toughen the delicate interdigital skin on the feet of hunting dogs. I have no idea how it works on dogs, but it works well on my feet.
>
> The formula: 30 cubic centimeters tincture of benzoin, 30 grams alum, 30 grams tannic acid, 10 cubic centimeters balsam of Peru and eight ounces petroleum jelly.
>
> I smear this mixture very liberally on my toes, then carefully roll my socks over the mess.

TIGHT SHOES

Q: After a few miles of running, my toes always blister and begin to take on the appearance of shredded wheat. Painful! My shoes seem tight fitting. One shoe salesman advised me to buy loose-fitting shoes to take the pressure off the toes. Another said to stay with tight-fitting shoes because "sliding around" can cause blisters, too. What would your advice be?

A: I like plenty of room upfront. However, most runners—like basketball players—wear shoes a size too small. I suggest you get a size larger (you can always wear an extra pair of anklets).

BLACK TOENAILS

Q: After any distance race, I end up with at least four black toenails which eventually are replaced but mean sore toes for some time. How can I save my toenails?

A: Black nails are due to hemorrhage under the nails. The cause is usually shoes a size too small or jamming of the toes from slippage (which can occur with larger shoes).

I have heard that Dr. Scholl's foam toe caps are sometimes a help. A reader told me he cured a chronic problem of blood blisters by using the toe caps. Even though they reduced the toe space in the shoe, he was able to run a marathon without difficulty.

CHAFING

Q: I have recently increased my mileage and have encountered a painful problem: chafing between the legs. I have tried Vaseline; it works, but can you suggest a less messy way?

A: Vaseline, messy as it is, is the answer. It is a staple in every runner's ditty bag. I use it liberally over any exposed area in winter running and to prevent chafing anyplace at all times.

BOILS

Q: For approximately nine months, I've been developing boils or carbuncles. I developed four under my right armpit, three on my left thigh, one on my left calf and several in the groin area.

I have been to a doctor. He performed a blood test to see if there was excessive sugar. The results were negative. He prescribd Tri-Sulfa antibiotic which helped kill the infection. I thought it was all over until I recently developed some more.

What is my running doing to this? I'm presently training lightly.

A: Recurrent boils occur in hair-bearing areas in susceptible people. The critical factor is the number of staphylococcus organisms in a given area. This can be reduced by thorough washing followed by liberal applications of rubbing alcohol to all hair-bearing areas. Reduction of irritation is also helpful.

Don't wear tight-fitting clothes over the area.

Boils occur in series, and the object is to break the cycle by preventing the next one. Use of anti-staphylococcus penicillin is sometimes indicated, and use of a staph toxoid has occasionally been successful.

I see no need to stop running while you have these. Physical activity (except for the sweating) does not seem to be a factor.

FEVER BLISTERS

Q: What can I do to avoid getting fever blisters when running? I get them on the upper lip after I have pushed a little hard during a race. It is more likely to occur at distances of 6-10 miles.

A: Fever blisters, or herpes simplex, are caused by a virus which can be reactivated by stress. In your case, the race is sufficient stress to produce the fever blister. I have heard of one professor who would get fever blisters only when he delivered a lecture on one particular subject, apparently a topic that he didn't quite command.

ITCHING

Q: About a year ago, after running I developed severe itching which was intense and felt all over my body. My dermatologist says it best be ignored. I have no known allergies and no history of skin problems. No remedy has surfaced and I turn to you in desperation.

A: You have a physical allergy precipitated by exercise. Your dermatologist is probably right; the best thing to do, if possible, is to ignore it.

However, in your case this isn't possible. It has almost caused you to stop running and is now a major problem. You must investigate every possibility that may help.

Consider the possibility that there is an associated food allergy which may help trigger these attacks. If so, it is something you take daily. That generally eliminates offenders like chocolate, shellfish and melon. It leaves egg whites, milk, citrus fruit, wheat and peanut butter. Try stopping those in bulk. If you get better, you can begin adding them back one at a time.

Avoid hot drinks. Take a cold shower instead of a hot one. Lower the thermostat below 70 degrees.

Try antihistamines.

Be sure you are not overtraining. Exhaustion always accentuates allergies.

Finally, you might consider a long-acting steroid shot. This is not without complications, and you should discuss it thoroughly with your physician.

SHAVING

Q: I am a bit embarrassed to be writing to you about this subject, but it is something that's held my curiosity for quite some time now. I've noticed pictures of Frank Shorter and Dick Buerkle, among others, show no hair on their arms and legs. Do they shave them for to cut down air drag? Do you think this would be helpful?

A: I am not sure if there are runners that shave their legs for cosmetic reasons. However, I do know that some competitive runners have done it.

Dixon Farmer, who coaches in Washington, reported having some of his runners shave their bodies to improve performance. This had already been done in swimmers, of course, but not to any extent in runners.

According to Farmer, shaving had a beneficial effect—primarily psychological—on performance. You feel like running is easier, so it is. You feel as if you are running faster, so you do.

Whether it helps or not, the runners who have done it say it gives them an unusual but enjoyable feeling.

BATHING

Q: In your book, *Dr. Sheehan on Running,* you mention toweling off rather than showering after a run. You describe the difference between sweat glands and, in so many words, challenge runners to recognize our middle-class hangups. Well, I read it the first time and skipped most of what you said. I read it again and dismissed it as zany, and the third time thought you were being antisocial. Now, after trying it when time was extremely short, I am doing it. The point: Running friends don't believe it. Some have even suggested I look at my schedule to see if appointments are being cancelled or falling off. Would you present the whole idea again?

A: Coming from a generation of "Saturday night bathers," I can see no reason to waste time on showers during the week.

It is sweat that cleanses. We are baptized in our own water, a pure dilute salt solution which can be toweled off as readily as any water provided by our community. Sweat cleanses from the inside. It comes from places a shower will never reach.

I have it on good authority that people who have embarked on running programs have been able to give up the use of deodorants where previously showers had been of only transient assistance. So nervous sweat is what causes smell, and no runners of my acquaintance have that odor.

Chapter 32
Genito-Urinary System

Disorders of the genito-urinary system that occur in endurance athletes usually have much more psychological impact than medical. Passing blood in the urine is one of the most alarming events in a runner's life. The threat of infertility, however vague, can be quite threatening to a male runner, as can the stoppage of menstruation in a female.

Many of these genito-urinological problems have resisted adequate explanation for a long time, and many still do. However, we have learned the mechanism in some instances and have arrived at suitable methods of treatment.

The most frequent conditions seen in this system of the body are as follows:

• *Amenorrhea.* Female runners with extremely high mileage problems have noted that their periods stop or become infrequent. In most instances, these runners are trained down fine and have an unusually low per cent body fat.

Adolescents who get into heavy training regimens may note the same phenomenon. Here, the relationship is not quite so clear, because menstruation may be chancy at that age.

The cause is speculative. Undoubtedly, training has an effect on numerous hormones of the body concerned with ovulation, as it does on every other function. We know that stress and starvation have been proven to have a depressing effect on the menses. Long-distance running involves both.

This disturbance is apparently reversible. Decreasing time and intensity of workouts leads to resumption of regular periods.

Treatment: No treatment is needed and there are no long-range effects. However, in adolescents, the possibility of an associated delay in growth must be considered.

• *Dysmenorrhea.* Many women runners report having lower abdominal menstrual pain, sometimes radiating to the upper thighs, not associated with the menstrual cycle. These pains are precipitated by ordinary training runs anytime during the month. Similar pains have also been noted by women using IUDs for contraception.

Of course, dysmenorrhea of the usual type can be distressing for the dedicated runner. It has been shown that the physiological changes during the period do not affect performance. However, the pain can.

Treatment: Recently, anti-prostaglandin drugs have been found to have a satisfactory therapeutic effect on menstrual cramps. The most generally used is aspirin. However, the most effective in general use is Indocin.

I have been criticized for recommending such a potent drug for a minor problem. But in runners, there are no minor problems. Anything that hinders or prevents running, or removes the enjoyment is a catastrophe.

Use of Indocin sparingly in 25-50-milligram doses is usually quite beneficial. This is, of course, something to be done under the direction and care of a physician.

• *Pregnancy.* Here, as in many areas, the information must come from the runners themselves. The textbooks simply don't have the information.

One survey by Janet Heinonen showed that most women ran up to the last month. Some ran until the day of delivery. Apparently, aerobic running has no harmful effect on the pregnancy or the fetus.

It is essential that it be an uncomplicated pregnancy. Bleeding or other problems during the first trimester are an indication to stop running.

The question of competition is unresolved. I know of at least one world-class swimmer competing during pregnancy, and the likelihood is that many runners do. It seems highly unlikely that the brief oxygen starvation of such efforts has any detrimental effect on the fetus. But the question has been raised and must be considered.

Dr. Dorothy Harris, one of the most highly respected researchers in this field, has taken a conservative approach and suggests cessation of competitive running.

• *Infertility in males.* The possibility of male infertility brought on by distance running has been suggested by runners themselves. Several have written to me about lowered sperm counts in their attempts to have children.

Whether this is coincidence or directly caused is, of course, difficult to say. Whether runners have a higher incidence of infertility problems remains to be seen. (There have, incidentally, been no reports of decreased libido from running.)

Treatment, if a causal relation is established: Runners who want to father children will have to stop running until sperm counts rise to an acceptable range.

• *Prostatitis.* Runner or not, chronic prostatitis is a difficult disease to treat. Most runners with this difficulty say it seems to remain symptomatic as long as they run. However, one or two have reported that running has cured their problem.

I think it comes down to the fact that urologists find chronic prostatitis a disease they do not handle with any optimism. The runner has to go the full route of antibiotics, massages and sitz baths. Even then, it will be a question of accepting some amount of symptoms.

Treatment: Physician-directed antibiotics, massage, sitz baths.

• *Epididymitis:* Occasionally, runners get acute inflammation of the epididymis, a mass of tubes at the back of the testes. This may be secondary to prostatic infection and brought on by trauma either direct or due to running without a support. The course of treatment may be prolonged and the inflammation tends to recur.

Treatment: Usual urological treatment of physician-directed antibiotics, massage, sitz baths plus support. Occasionally, running must be stopped in order to allow symptoms to subside.

• *Blood in urine:* The passage of blood by runners has been recorded officially in medical texts going back to 1700. I am sure diligent search might discover references in Greek literature, Maimonides or Galen, if not others.

It wasn't, however, until May 1977, when a British naval surgeon reported 18 runners with this condition, that we learned the cause. Immediate cystoscopy uniformly discovered bruising of the bladder wall. These injuries clear rapidly, usually in 5-7 days, explaining why they had not been discovered before. The tests were done too late.

This delay is usual in studying such injuries. First, a urinalysis is done, then kidney X-rays and finally, because of reluctance on the part of the patient, a cystoscopy. The traditional discipline of the British naval service bypassed these amenities and went right to the core of the problem.

Prior to the British studies, innumerable runners had been subjected to innumerable investigatory procedures, all with normal results. Rarely, a non-running cause of hematuria was discovered. One runner of my acquaintance was discovered to have a kidney tumor. Another had a kidney stone.

But knowing the result (the bruise) still does not get to the cause. What was the mechanism of this bruising?

Dr. N. J. Blacklock suggests that it is due to an empty bladder. The lack of cushioning urine in the bladder allows it to impact on the pubic bone. To a man, his runners had taken inadequate fluids prior to the run.

Another suggestion is that a full colon contributes to the problem. I have a feeling both factors contribute.

I had a call from a man in Florida who ran at 6 a.m. without having a bowel movement on taking fluids. He bled almost daily. I also had a call on a summer day from a runner who had bled after a 10,000-meter run and had not taken fluids for six hours prior to the race.

Treatment: An empty colon and a partially full bladder seem to be the answer. Like many other conditions, the tendency to bruising may be idiosyncratic and then cyclical. So it probably affects susceptible people at susceptible times of the year, either due to exhaustion or allergies.

• *Hemoglobinuria and pigmenturia.* Not all red urine contains blood. It may be due to hemoglobin (or a result of breakdown of red cells); myoglobin (breakdown of muscle tissue); or to dyes and pigments in the urine or secondary to certain foods.

Hemoglobinuria is thought to be caused by impact shock on the blood cells at footstrike. The hemoglobin thus liberated filters through the kidney and colors the urine. It is essential, therefore, to obtain a specimen and differentiate these various types of pigmenturia.

Hemoglobinuria also tends to be cyclic. The cause of this is, again, unknown. There is probably some relation to the status of the auto-immune system. In other words, allergy, neuro-hormonal state and the homeostatic equilibrium are all factors.

Although alarming, hemoglobinuria is a relatively benign condition. The hemoglobin molecule is small and does not affect the kidneys. Also, the blood loss is infinitesimal.

Myoglobinuria, however, is a different story. This is a large molecule and can block the kidneys. The result can be a kidney shutdown, and the patient may need dialysis. Myoglobinuria is caused by severe, prolonged muscle effort (as in a marathon) with associated additional stress such as heat, humidity and dehydration. Usually, heat stroke is a concomitant event, although not necessarily so.

Some individuals may be susceptible because of some enzymatic deficiencies at the muscular level. Occasionally, runners who depleted for carbohydrate-loading reasons have subsequently had myoglobinuria. Fasting or high-protein diets may set a susceptible individual up for such an event.

Urine may also be colored by bladder medications such as Pyridium or by foods.

Treatment of hemoglobinuria: Reduction of shock by appropriate shoes. Add Spenco inserts. Restrict running to grass. Reduce training program to every other day. Eliminate allergens. Increase nap time.

Myoglobinuria: Prevention of dehydration is essential. Minor amounts of myoglobin can be noted after prolonged runs, but apparently hydration is the chief weapon. Also, general rules for handling heat must be followed.

If you are going to carbohydrate load, do not deplete, just load.

• *Microscopic hematuria and proteinuria.* The finding of microscopic hematuria is very frequent in runners. One study done after a race in Oregon showed that 17% of the runners had microscopic blood in the urine. Protein also is fairly frequently present. Both conditions clear immediately and are not seen under other conditions.

Since the blood is invisible, it concerns the physician more than the runner. It is of such widespread occurrence, with no known complications or after-effects, that the condition should only be of academic interest. Unfortunately, well-meaning physicians occasionally issue precautionary statements, thereby creating problems where none exist.

Treatment: None needed. Such findings are physiological and commensurate with the time intensity and cardiovascular state (hydration, blood volume, etc.) of the runner.

KIDNEYS

Q: Several years ago, I had one of my kidneys removed. I am wondering if this would in any way affect my performance or ability as a runner.

A: I see no reason why having only one kidney will affect your performance. You should avoid contact sports like football or hockey. But running is not only a safe and acceptable activity, it is also one which does not depend on two kidneys.

VASECTOMY

Q: Several runners over 40 have reported complications (bleeding) following vasectomies. All of them run substantial distances. Is there a higher proportion of such complications among runners than in the population at large? Is there any reason there might be more such problems among runners?

A: My urological colleague tells me there is a 7% complication rate after vasectomies, mostly bleeding and infection.

Neither of these, however, is a serious problem, and both can be handled easily. One specialist told me that he does the vasec-tomies as an office procedure and allows runners to run the next day.

My expert tells me it is his surgical experience that fit people heal, if anything, more quickly. As to slow recovery from ab-dominal surgery, my experience is the direct opposite. I ran 10 days after my gall bladder surgery and competed in a five-mile race within three weeks of the operation date.

MENSTRUAL MISERY

Q: Female readers would be interested to know if so-called pre-menstrual tension causes any measurable physiological ef-fects which could influence aerobic and anaerobic running per-formance. My own observations indicate that on "those bad days," workouts involving speed and anaerobic endurance are the most difficult—my intervals are slower than usual, and I tend to fade out as soon as I get winded. Long, slow runs, on the other hand, provide relatively little trouble and can even make me feel better. Have there been any studies on this sub-ject?

A: The pre-menstrual days are usually marked by pain, headache, bloating and, in younger women, skin eruptions. The main observable phenomenon is fluid retention.

In one Finnish study of 1000 women, sports participation sig-nificantly reduced signs and symptoms of pre-menstrual prob-lems. But other than that, no research is indexed in the litera-ture.

I know there is passing mention to athletic performance dur-ing "those days" in articles in the popular press. My memory is that Olympic medals have been won and world records broken during this time.

Your own experience suggests that anaerobic activity can suffer during that time. I doubt that the exact mechanism for that would be known even to exercise physiologists. The experts have more to learn from the athlete than vice-versa—especially in the field of women's sports.

NURSING MOTHERS

Q: I have been nursing my baby five months now and am planning on attempting a marathon this summer. Before the baby came, I ran, swam and biked without becoming fatigued. But now running and swimming seem very exhausting. Must I sacrifice my physical exercise to nurse?

A: Nursing does cause easy fatigue. I have that on good authority from some women in my family. Part of it may be the size and weight of the breasts, but it seems to be more than that.

Perhaps you should experiment with exercising immediately before or after nursing, and notice the difference. In any case, treat yourself as an experiment of one.

WOMEN AND IRON

Q: I can't run more than 2½ miles without having a run-down feeling. I read Joan Ullyot's book (*Women's Running*) and she suggests taking 100 milligrams of ferrous gluconate with each meal for 4-6 weeks, which I did.

But then I read other things that say some people don't absorb inorganic iron correctly, and it somehow can go to your liver or other organs, or to your joints—which means disaster. So I cut back on the iron supplement, and now I'm back to my usual fatigue and slow pace. I had a blood test that showed I'm not anemic.

I'm 46 years old and have been running about three years. Is there any way to tell if your body is not absorbing the iron correctly or if you are getting too much? I did feel much better after using the iron supplement. Does this mean I should continue with the iron?

A: I'm inclined to agree with taking the medication. You probably need the 100 milligrams daily. That did make you feel better, and if it does again, there can be no doubt. That's the answer.

Need for iron is not necessarily shown by a blood test. The marrow stores (and with them the enzyme systems) may be depleted while the blood count is still normal. Only a bone marrow study will tell.

Other deficiencies may, of course, be present. Thyroid, B-12, folic acid or other, more obscure supplemental vitamins may be needed.

Go back to your iron. If you feel no better, test your thyroid and other levels, such as folic acid and B-12.

Chapter 33
Headaches, Hemorrhoids, Etc.

HEARING

Q: I've noticed that during long or hard runs, my power of hearing decreases. When I breathe or talk, it sounds hollow or like an echo. What causes this? Is it a common occurrence?

A: I think your hearing loss results from blockage of the eustachian tube. This passage connects the nasal passage to the middle ear to allow equalization of pressure. It is the reason you can swallow and clear your ears when you go up and down in an elevator.

Apparently, prolonged and intense breathing can cause swelling around the opening in the nasal passage and block it. I have experienced this blocked feeling plus a sensation of water in my ears after particularly strenuous or competitive runs.

Use of a nasal spray before or immediately after running may help. I get relief from bending over and holding my head down for a few seconds. Swallowing with the nose pinched is sometimes helpful.

VISION LOSS

Q: I believe it has been reported by long-distance runners that in the final stages of a marathon a temporary loss of peripheral vision may take place. Is there any danger of permanent damage from this and, if so, how can a runner avoid it?

A: The loss of peripheral vision is a temporary phenomenon probably secondary to diminished oxygen supply. Pilots are urged to use oxygen over 5000 feet on night flights to improve their peripheral vision. Runners probably experience a similar situation.

In extreme cases of oxygen deficiency, retinal hemorrhages can occur. This has been reported in mountain climbers. These individuals, however, are climbing to 14,000 feet and over. In some instances, the damage was permanent, in others reversible.

I know of only one instance where a marathoner was left with a visual-field defect after collapsing in a marathon. As always, it is a matter of listening to your body and not continuing when the physiology is coming apart.

DIZZINESS

Q: I frequently feel dizzy when standing up from a squatting or stooping position. Is this something to be concerned about? I am 45, weigh 151 pounds, 5'10" tall, blood pressure 110/80, pulse down to 42.

A: You are describing a phenomenon called orthostatic hypotension—i.e., a drop in blood pressure immediately on assuming a standing position. It should go up.

I have experienced this just about when I am peaking out (or overtraining), so it appears to be a near-exhaustion symptom. At any rate, I view it as such and usually cut back on the frequency and intensity of training.

In my practice, it also appears to be an exhaustion phenomenon, and patients who experience this usually have this feeling 4-6 weeks before it disappears. The medical explanation is relative adrenal insufficiency (which Hans Seyle defines as a failure of adaptation).

HEADACHES

Q: My vascular headaches disappeared when I started marathon training one year ago. Recently, after my best marathon, I had a severe three-day headache. Can I expect more? What can I do to prevent this?

A: People with vascular headaches inherit a lifelong tendency to this disorder. They can recur after months or years of freedom from symptoms. Some experts have suggested that certain foods can pull the trigger leading to an attack if you are allergic to them. Chocolate is frequently cited as a causative agent. Recent research has focused on several types of foods known to precipitate attacks and has given rise to the following dietary suggestions:

1. Avoid alcohol, particularly red wines and champagne.

2. Avoid aged or strong cheese, particularly cheddar cheese.

3. Avoid chicken livers, pickled herring, canned figs, pods of broad beans.

4. Use monosodium glutamate sparingly.

5. Avoid cured meats such as hotdogs, bacon, ham or salami if these can be demonstrated to evoke vascular headache.

6. Eat three well-balanced meals a day. Avoid skipping meals, prolonged fasting or eating excessive amounts of carbohydrates at any single meal.

You will have to keep a food diary and write down all food eaten for 36 hours before the headache. After two or three headaches, the recurrence of some specific food item may incriminate it as the causative agent.

Vascular headache can also occur from carbon monoxide exposure. The possibility of excessive carbon monoxide exposure should also be considered, especially if your marathon went through areas of heavy traffic.

Q: After suffering chronic post-training headaches, I decided to increase my intake of potassium. It worked. How can I get potassium in foods for extra protection?

A: Every experience helps. What worked for you may work for others. Many researchers have stressed potassium loss secondary to daily strenuous exercise in hot, humid conditions.

It makes sense. We were originally herbivores. The body was made to hang on to salt very tenaciously. However, if anything, potassium excretion increases with exercise.

The resultant symptoms may be anything from muscle cramps to exhaustion to kidney failure. Headache may be due to this gradual depletion as well.

As you discovered, there is little or no need for extra salt. Usually, the amount of salt in the ordinary diet is enough. But we should probably make an effort to get extra potassium. Fruit juices are excellent. A low-salt meat stock soup is also a prime source. Commercial potassium preparations are available, the most palatable I think is K-lyte, an effervescent powder.

PINCHED NERVE

Q: I now run about 25-30 miles a week and generally feel fine except for one strange pain. After about three miles, I get a shocking, tingling sensation in my right wrist, just behind the thumb. This happens when my right arm swings down as my left foot hits the ground. I have tried moving my right arm around and stretching it now and then while running, but this doesn't do much. Is there anything I can do?

A: Such pain indicates a pinched nerve, either at the wrist (carpal tunnel), shoulder (outlet syndrome) or neck spine (radiculitis). You will have to see a physician and have him tell you which. I would recommend you see an orthopedic surgeon. In any case, it is more of a nuisance than anything else.

HEMORRHOIDS

Q: I developed a hemorrhoid right after the New York City marathon. I never had trouble of this sort before, and now I am having difficulty getting rid of it. Must I stop running to cure it?

A: Hemorrhoids are only incidentally due to long-distance running. They occur when a runner delays having a bowel movement, or when abnormal constipation results from low fluid intake and a low-fiber diet.

The classic sport for hemorrhoids is mountain climbing. When you are at 15,000 feet and the winds are 25 knots, you are likely to put off a bowel movement until the following summer. That's when hemorrhoids and anal fissures occur.

I have had some correspondence with runners who had their hemorrhoids cured by running. One runner who had been using a suppository daily with not much effect before he began running reported an almost complete cure after three months into a running program. This is apparently due to the increased bowel peristalsis that takes place during running. This corrected his constipation.

Hemorrhoids respond to answering the call when it comes and insuring daily bulky movements with a high-fiber diet.

VARICOSE VEINS

Q: I am 30 years old, and during my last pregnancy developed a varicose vein. Because of this, my leg aches, but I want to start running with my husband. A doctor advised taking vitamin C and wearing support hose. Will this help my problem?

A: Movement is good for varicose veins. Running is no hazard. I would encourage you to develop a smooth, relatively short stride and avoid excessive up and down movement.

I'm not sure the vitamin C does much for veins, but the support hose is a good idea. Also, avoid excessive standing.

GOUT

Q: I have seen no articles on the gouty runner. What is the effect of running with these symptoms?

A: The common feature of people with gout is an excessive uric acid pool in the body. Clinical gout occurs when urate crystals deposit from supersaturated body fluids.

The exact mechanisms that cause this are unknown. Clinicians have thought, rightly or wrongly, that starvation, great effort or excessive intake of purines in food can precipitate an attack. Recently, relative adrenal insufficiency has been considered a trigger factor. The occurrence of acute gout soon after major surgery would seem to confirm this.

My opinion is that gouty runners have two types of gout reactions to running. The first is muscular and joint pain due to an approaching fatigue state. These pains are not associated with swelling or tenderness. They are also in joints and tissues unrelated to running.

The second gout problem is the tendinitis that Canadian researchers have described. But I have a different interpretation of this. Here, the gouty reaction is in the tendon, joint, fascia or whatever, that is bearing the brunt of some structural imbalance.

In both instances, the essential treatment is physiological: (a) reducing training if a fatigue state exists; (b) restoring structural balance where a specific area is under stress (using foot supports, for instance).

A runner with gout unrelated to running should be on the usual regimen of drugs, diets and fluids as recommended by his physician.

DIABETES

Q: A 14-year-old patient of mine with diabetes plans to participate in both track and cross-country. In cross-country, he would be competing over the three-mile distance. What problems do you anticipate with a diabetic in distance running, both in training and competition, in regard to utilization of glycogen stores and possible insulin reactions? How should his diet be modified?

A: Long-distance running puts a drain on available glycogen in a diabetic. This action can have especially serious effects unless prepared for adequately.

First, it appears that such glycogen stores are not threatened in runs of six miles or less. However, repeated daily heavy training schedules can cause chronic depletion. This suggests that his training schedule should allow for replenishment of glycogen reserves by having his alternate days extremely light. In addition, his glycogen supply should not be challenged acutely by runs over six miles—at least not until he has found a definite and predictable pattern of response.

As to insulin and diet: (1) he should reduce his insulin to one-half on the days of racing or hard training; (2) he should have a high-protein meal before running; (3) sugar and orange juice should be available at the running area, which should be a small area until his pattern of response is established; (4) the major problem is maintenance of glycogen stores which can be done with a high-carbohydrate diet on easy running days.

HERNIAS

Q: I have just had my hernia repaired with a 30-minute

operation done under local anesthesia. I am ready to go home after 72 hours. I understand you have a similar problem but resist surgery. Why?

A: My hernias have become a medical scandal. Surgeons just will not take seriously my decision to retain them. The fact that I am a physician who should know that all hernias must be repaired makes my statement doubly amusing or irritating, depending on their mood.

It gave me great pleasure, therefore, to read in the *Annals of Internal Medicine* that I might be on the right track. Someone took the trouble to trace the natural history of groin hernias and the fate of patients, depending upon whether or not they had been operated upon.

Before informing you of the result, I will tell you that the surgeons' usual response to my report that my two hernias don't bother me, so why be operated upon is, "It will strangulate and you will be in real trouble." When surgeons say "real trouble," they mean the worst.

But what did the research on hernias reveal? Well, that people who resisted surgery lived longer than those who had the hernias repaired.

So I'll wait. It's true a 30-minute operation has some appeal. But I suspect I am made of the kind of material that would immediately come apart again, with another hernia replacing the one that had been repaired.

AFTER SURGERY

In the past, I have received many questions about athletic activity after major abdominal surgery. I can now answer from personal experience.

The ninth day after my gall bladder was removed, I rode a bike without difficulty. The following day in a fit of depression, I jogged a mile. Within two weeks, I was back to six miles a day. Less than three weeks from surgery, I ran a five-mile race. At no time did I have pain. The race felt no different from usual, except I was running about one minute a mile slower.

After six weeks, I was running only 10-15 seconds a mile slower than normal. And after about two months, I seemed to be running normally again.

The runner apparently can tolerate returning to activity at an early date. He will, however, take some time to return to competitive form. Fatigue comes on more easily, and I found it necessary to limit running to 15 minutes (or even resting) on alternate days.

My surgeon, incidentally, thought I was nuts. It may take time to rewrite the book. After all, I'm in my 50s and not very special. Recovering after surgery should be an easy process for anyone in his prime.

CANCER

Q: I recently read an article in a journal not related to sports medicine that cancer formation in cells grown in a test tube is prevented by exposure to oxygenated hemoglobin. The authors postulate that lowered oxygen content may play a role in producing a cancer. The question that arises is this: Do runners have less cancer because of the increased oxygenation of their tissues?

A: It has long been the contention of Dr. Ernst van Aaken that distance running does protect runners for the reason you describe. However, another recent report shows that distance runners may have *more* cancer than the average population. This is the thesis of a study reported in the *Journal of Sports Medicine and Physical Fitness*, June 1975.

Whether running makes a difference one way or the other, I can't say. But I can say that anyone who is running just to prevent heart attacks or cancer should be casting around for a more satisfying activity. Life is too short to waste it on such practical things as fitness for its own sake.

PART NINE:
THE ENVIRONMENT

"It is not enough to have guts.
You must listen to them."

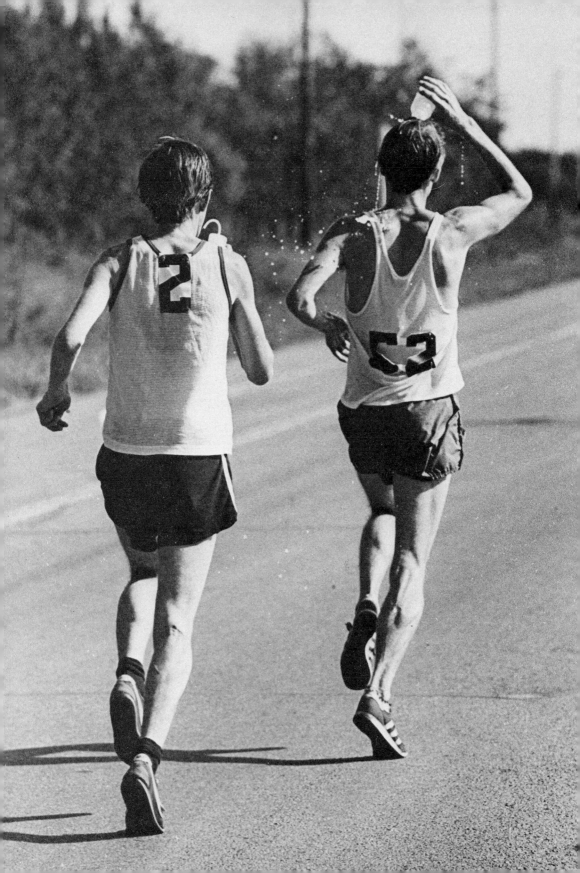

Chapter 34
Listening to Yourself

The animal moves through this life with certainty. He appears to know exactly why he is here, where he is going and what to do about it. The animal gets in trouble only when it accepts domesticated goals or civilized lifestyles. The horse may die from running in a race. The pampered pet grows gross and dependent. Disaster occurs when human reasoning replaces animal instinct.

"Man is surely farther from the truth about life," wrote James Thurber, "than any other animal this side of the ladybug."

At the 1973 Boston Marathon, only 700 of the 1400 starters certified as being capable of running a marathon in 3:30 actually did so. Almost a dozen ended in hospitals with exhaustion, and hundreds of others walked in long after the officials had departed. Again, it was a case of inadequate human knowledge replacing the fundamental intuitions of the body, of man-made goals and predetermined pace taking precedence over the subconscious perceptions the runner gets from his body.

At Boston that year, the problem was not simply the 26.2-mile distance. It was distance compounded by heat. Patriot's Day came up unseasonably warm. At 79 degrees, it was the hottest April 16 in the history of Boston.

Optimum temperature for long-distance running is 40-45 degrees. Each additional 10 degrees makes the course run longer, just as a golf course plays longer in certain weather. And the best way to handle this additional load is attention to the three

P's: *Preparation, Pace and Perspiration.*

Experienced runners like Ron Daws have found they can prepare their body for hot weather. Still, prepared or not, the body cannot pursue endurance runs in hot weather at a cold-weather pace. Part of the oxygen capacity of the system is necessarily given over to heat dissipation and withdrawn from the work output.

The pace, then, is crucial. The runner's body must accept all this confusing meteorological data and come up with the pace-of-the-day. That pace is no less than the maximum pace that can be held indefinitely. That, in essence, is what the ultimate experimental animal, the human being, is attempting to discover in this ultimate human experiment, the Boston Marathon.

This pace, however, is also determined by how the runner handles his perspiration balance. Perspiration must be completely replaced, and to do this you must start early. Some runners go from one cultist idea to another: drink nothing; do not drink before the 10th mile; drink only thus and such.

But the body tells you the truth and that is to take as much water as you can get, as soon as you can get it. The body seems to know early on that the runner will sweat out 4-5 quarts of water, will lose quantities of salt and potassium and will have a rise in temperature to 104 degrees.

Relying on his instincts, the runner begins to know what levers to trip, what trough to feed from. He lets his body take over. He listens and learns.

Most of all, the runner learns to listen. Having gone through the peril of the Boston, he now recognizes that his survival comes from within. The danger is always from without: man-made goals, book-learned pace, hypothetical diets and so much more that has to do with lifestyle, values, guilt and compulsions.

The runner realizes that he becomes more rational as he becomes more animal.

"The finer mysteries of life," Thurber added, "may be comprehended only through instinct." To be a man, it is not enough to have guts. You must listen to them.

Chapter 35
Heat and Cold

A HOT RACE

We had a five-mile race in our town. It was a hot, muggy day with a bright sun, little cloud cover and virtually no wind—a day to make use of every trick I knew about handling heat.

Many runners, I am sure, did not even think of the day as hot. For them, the temperature of 69 degrees was seasonable for a day in mid-June. However, it was the humidity that was important. At 79%, it was high enough to elevate almost any temperature to a dangerous level.

When the heat stress is that severe, almost any race is a long race. Two years earlier, we had three runners hospitalized with temperatures over 106 after a five-mile race. All three had been training and were apparently acclimatized to heat.

The key to heat stress is how much fluid your body loses in sweat in a given period of time. The body adapts to heat by sweating and the cooling effect of its evaporation from the skin. The amount of sweat can be almost unbelievable.

A friend of mine who dropped out of a very hot Boston Marathon at the 14-mile mark discovered that he had lost 12 pounds, or five quarts of sweat. He was fortunate not to have suffered an acute heat syndrome. Loss of 5% water weight can lead occasionally to catastrophe.

The object, then, is to minimize this loss—to take plenty of fluids even before the race, as well as during it. The most important ingredient is water. Only secondarily should we worry

257

about what is in it.

For an hour or so before our five-mile race, I drank fluids, water at times, but mostly iced tea in quantities that eventually made me urinate. Only that way could I be assured I was in my normal hydrated state.

By now it was about 15 minutes to go, and they began giving us the instructions for the race. There was to be, they said, one water station. It would be at the three-mile mark.

They were wrong. There were to be two water stations. One was on the starting line. Right there, I took six ounces of water and six ounces of iced tea. I was now ready for the first three miles—more ready, I suspected, than anyone else standing there awaiting the gun.

The race was the hot one the temperature and the humidity promised. Fortunately, we ran on tree-lined streets and were in the shade almost the entire way, so radiant heat was not a factor.

At the halfway mark, I was struggling to stay with a group that was ticking off six-minute miles. Nearing the water station, I could feel them drawing away from me. I was beginning to lose ground to them and to the clock. Then came the hose and the tables with the cups and people handing them out. Most of those ahead of me took a quick drink, hardly more than a gulp, and went on. Some never even looked as they passed by.

When I reached this relief station, I stopped and stood there drinking. I downed two full six-ounce cups, doused another over my head and then set out in pursuit. They had gained about 50 yards on me. But if the rules of physiology held up, I would catch them before the finish.

Water not only saves, you see, it also insures maximum performance. Keeping your fluid level normal also keeps your blood volume normal. That is what allows you to run efficiently. Passing up the water not only sets you up for a heat stroke, it does something worse, it makes you run badly.

And that was the way it was. Coming into that last mile, I had made up the 50 yards I had lost. I was back in the pack and knew now I was the strongest among them. It was just a matter of being tough on that hill, and then I sprinted home with no one near me. My time was just over 31 minutes for the five, comparable to my cold-weather times.

Two minutes later, a runner half my age crossed the line and collapsed. He was taken to the hospital, given two quarts of fluid by vein and subsequently a quart by mouth before his circulation came back into the normal range.

What had happened was that he had taken no fluid before the race. He had heard, he said, conflicting stories about taking water. So he had rinsed his mouth out and then run the race. Had he stopped at the water station? "Just for a mouthful." So he had run a five-mile race in heat and humidity with the protection of one ounce of water. The result was near-disaster.

It was also instructive that he had felt no thirst. And that at no time had he suspected he was in difficulty. Heat is really a silent killer. The victim is down for the count before any warning comes.

The deficit in water begins at the gun, and for that reason we must begin to make it up in advance. Playing catch-up is not a game that works in hot-weather running.

Still, as my race demonstrated, there is a way to make hot-weather running safe, efficient and even enjoyable. Running has always been a sport where effort pays off. Training has time and again made up for limited talent. It is also a sport where intelligence counts, where physiology works, where science is helpful, and where understanding what is happening to your body can make the difference between talking about heat stroke and having one.

KEEP COOL

Living may be easy in the summertime, but distance running is not. Summer heat and humidity hamper performance, even threaten health and life to such a degree that the American College of Sports Medicine issued the following "position statement on prevention of heat injuries during distance running":

> Since it is likely that distance running enthusiasts will continue to sponsor races under adverse heat conditions, specific steps should be taken to minimize the health threats which accompany such endurance events.
> Fluid ingestion during prolonged running has been shown effectively to reduce rectal temperature and minimize dehydration. Although most

competitors consume fluids during races that exceed 1-1½ hours, many events do not offer or some runners do not take drinks until an hour or more has passed. Under such limitations, the competitor is certain to accumulate a large body water deficit before any fluids would be ingested.

To make the problem more complex, most runners are unable to judge the volume of fluids they consume during competition (and usually don't take enough to satisfy their needs). It seems obvious that the practices that prohibit fluid administration during distance running preclude any benefits that may be gained from this practice.

Runners who attempt to consume large volumes of a sugar solution during competition complain of gastric discomfort (fullness) and an inability to consume fluids after the first few feedings. Generally speaking, most runners drink solutions containing 5-20 grams of sugar per 100 milliliters of water. Although saline is rapidly emptied from the stomach, the addition of even small amounts of sugar can drastically impair the rate of gastric emptying. During exercise in the heat, carbohydrate supplementation is of secondary importance, and the sugar content of the oral feedings should be minimized.

Based on research findings and current rules governing distance running competition, it is the position of the American College of Sports Medicine that:

1. Distance races above 10 miles should *not* be conducted when the wetbulb temperature-globe temperature exceeds 82 F. (The weather bureau uses the THI—temperature humidity index. The equivalent THI is 79. Call the local weather station for readings.)

2. During periods of the year when the daylight drybulb temperature often exceeds 80 F., distance races should be conducted before 9 a.m. or after 4 p.m.

3. It is the responsibility of race sponsors to provide fluids which contain small amounts of sugar (glucose) and electrolytes (sodium and potassium).

4. Runners should be encouraged to ingest fluids frequently during competition and to consume 400-500 milliliters (13-17 ounces) of fluid 10-15 minutes before competition.

5. In light of the high sweating rates and body temperatures during distance running in the heat, race sponsors should provide "water stations" at 2-2½ mile intervals for all races of 10 miles or more.

6. Runners should be instructed in how to recognize the early warning symptoms that precede heat injury. Recognition of symptoms, cessation of running and proper treatment can prevent heat injury. Early warning symptoms include the following: pilo-erection on chest and upper arms, chilling, throbbing, pressure in the heat, unsteadiness, nausea and dry skin.

7. Race sponsors should make prior arrangements with medical personnel for the care of cases of heat injury. Responsible and informed

personnel should supervise each feeding station. Organizational personnel should reserve the right to stop runners who exhibit clear signs of
heat stroke or heat exhaustion.

It is the position of the American College of Sports Medicine that
policies established by local, national and international sponsors of distance running events should adhere to these guidelines. Failure to
adhere to these guidelines may jeopardize the health of competitors
through heat injury.

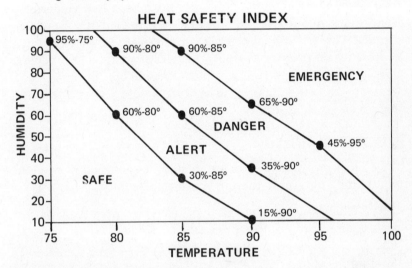

DEHYDRATION

The danger of dehydration continues to be underestimated.
Loss of more than 3% body weight puts the runner in a dangerous position. Prevention of heat problems is best done by con-
suming adequate amounts of *cool* water, according to Carl
Gisolfi of the University of Iowa.

Gisolfi gave runners running in a temperature of 91 degrees
F. 6.6 ounces of cold (50 degrees F.) water every 20 minutes.
This proved more effective than 6.6 ounces at body temperature. Sponging face and trunk for two minutes every 20 minutes
with towels soaked in 50-degree water was ineffective.

SWEAT SUITS

Q: I purchased a rubber sweat suit last year, and my friends
say I'm killing myself. But I feel that I replace most of the salt
and liquid after a run. Do I have to give up the suit and losing
weight?

A: The only purpose of a rubber suit would be to acclimate you to the heat. The suit puts stress on your heat dissipating system and makes it work better. After 10-14 days, you will sweat more readily and copiously. Your sweat will have a diminished salt content. And your circulatory system will get rid of heat more efficiently.

Does it help you lose weight? The rubber suit won't do this. Also, since it does cause significant heat retention, you should be cautious about pushing yourself into one of the heat syndromes. This could be dangerous in the summer. In the winter, it presents no problem unless you lose more than 3% of your body weight during a run. If you continue to use the suit in cool weather, take 10 ounces or so of fluid before you run to offset any excessive fluid loss.

WINTER TRAINING

Q: How do runners manage to stay in condition during the winter and run a marathon in the spring?

A: While long training pays off in good marathon performance, an adequate marathon can be run off relatively small mileage. Art Coolidge placed sixth at Boston (in 1971) after devoting his winter to cross-country skiing. He used a mere six weeks to tune up for the marathon.

You can probably run a creditable marathon working out one hour a day, five days a week, with a long run on Sundays. These requirements do not seem excessive whatever the weather conditions.

I've heard Canadians put on so much gear they looked like visitors from another planet when they get on the roads. It doesn't seem likely that your winter weather exceeds that of Guelph, Winnipeg, Fairbanks or other places where people run outdoors regularly.

Forty per cent of heat is lost through the head. Attention to that area with a ski mask and thermal underwear along with a few layers of light gear followed by a nylon shell will handle any weather.

After establishing a winter base, a few races at 10-15 miles in the six weeks before the big race are a great help to performance.

FREEZING THE LUNGS

"Freezing of the lungs," an oft-expressed worry of coaches and runners in very cold weather, does not occur. Carl Gisolfi, the University of Iowa physiologist who has centered his research on the reaction of the human body to heat and cold, says there is no evidence of cold injury to the larynx or bronchi.

According to Gisolfi, when air is inspired at 40 degrees below 0 F., it is already at 50-60 above when tested in the mouth. He suggests, however, that the extreme dryness of cold air may lead to cracking and bleeding of the respiratory passages. This may account for the fact that Arctic explorers frequently cough up blood for a few hours after heavy exertion.

WIND-CHILL READINGS								
Temperature (Farenheit)								
Calm	40	35	30	25	20	15	10	5
Equivalent Chill Temperature								
5	35	30	25	20	15	10	5	0
10	30	20	15	10	5	0	-10	-15
15	25	15	10	0	-5	-10	-20	-25
20	20	10	5	0	-10	-15	-25	-30
25	15	10	0	-5	-15	-20	-30	-35
30	10	5	0	-10	-20	-25	-30	-40
35	10	5	-5	-10	-20	-25	-35	-40
40	10	0	-5	-15	-20	-30	-35	-45

WIND (M.P.H.)

Little Danger   Increasing Danger

(Farenheit)								
0	-5	-10	-15	-20	-25	-30	-35	-40
Equivalent Chill Temperature								
-5	-10	-15	-20	-25	-30	-35	-40	-45
-20	-25	-35	-40	-45	-50	-60	-65	-70
-30	-40	-45	-50	-60	-65	-70	-80	-85
-35	-45	-50	-60	-65	-75	-80	-85	-95
-45	-50	-60	-65	-75	-80	-90	-95	-105
-50	-55	-65	-70	-80	-85	-95	-100	-105
-50	-60	-65	-75	-80	-90	-100	-105	-115
-55	-60	-70	-75	-85	-95	-100	-110	-115

Increasing Danger   Great Danger
(Flesh may freeze   (Flesh may freeze
within one minute)   within 30 seconds)

Chapter 36
Pollution and Altitude

DIRTY AIR

One of the major concerns of urban runners is air pollution. They wonder whether running in the city can cause more harm than good. They worry that pollutants in the atmosphere may cause immediate and long-term harmful effects on the body. The following discussion may help clear the air.

Q: What is air pollution?

A: The definition of air pollution varies from city to city, and from country to country. There is, you see, no agreement on what levels of what pollutants are dangerous. There are, therefore, no U.S. national standards for air pollution.

In general, when you hear that the air quality is acceptable or unacceptable, the reporters are talking about either particulate matter—sulfur oxides and smoke (black suspended material)—or ozone, the major ingredient in petrochemical smog. Carbon monoxide is almost always at the same level and does not enter into the rating.

Q: Are there standards of pollution rating that you subscribe to?

A: I like the criteria suggested by the World Health Organization. Air quality, according to them, depends on two factors.

The first is development of symptoms, of eye and respiratory irritation. The second is a decrease in visibility. When these occur, air quality is bad. As these increase, air quality gets worse.

I am a firm believer that the body knows when things are going wrong. Nature does not cause trouble without a warning. If the air pollution is bad, nature will let us know.

Q: What about carbon monoxide? That causes no eye or respiratory symptoms, or any change in visibility, yet it certainly can be dangerous.

A: Carbon monoxide is no threat to the runner. It merely combines with the hemoglobin in the blood and diminishes our ability to utilize oxygen. What it does, therefore, is simulate high-altitude training. Under high-carbon-monoxide conditions, you have about the same amount of available oxygen as you would if you were running in Denver. If you are already in Denver, then it is as if you were running in Leadville.

Running in traffic, then, is the poor man's method of training in Colorado. If, however, you are still concerned, you should run to the windward of auto traffic, stay a few yards away on the sidewalk, and avoid intersections where cars are stopped for any length of time.

Q: Has air pollution been demonstrated to impair running performance?

A: Yes. Studies done in high concentrations of ozone or petrochemical smog have shown decreased performance. Some of this work was done in California. Other researchers in Japan have come to much the same conclusion.

Ozone seems to be the one pollutant proven to decrease lung function. Fortunately, significant concentrations of petrochemical smog are found only in a few areas. Most of the United States is spared this problem. Chief victims of this pollutant are runners in the Los Angeles area.

Q: Are there any long-term effects of exposure to ozone?

A; Oddly enough, people seem to adapt to long-term exposure, so that the effects of the ozone diminish rather than increase. In a study done comparing the reaction of Canadians and nativeborn Angelenos to ozone, it was discovered that similar concentrations of the gas caused significantly more symptoms in the Canadians.

Q; How about the other pollutants?

A: It has been established that air pollution has an aggravating role on chronic respiratory disease. In other words, if you already have a chronic respiratory ailment, you will have more frequent and more serious problems with it.

However, its effect on causing emphysema and bronchitis is less certain. Nor can it be implicated as a causal agent in lung cancer. There is no comparison with the far more harmful effects of smoking, which also potentiates and amplifies bad effects of air pollution.

Q: Is there any defense against this air pollution?

A: In cities where there is little petrochemical smog, the main pollutants are smoke and sulfur dioxides. Theoretically, humidity increases the effects of these particles on the lungs, whereas rain actually washes the air. Heat also is said to increase the toxicity of these substances. It seems to me, therefore, that early morning or late evening may be times that pollution lessens.

Q: What about wearing a mask?

A: My friend Vin Chiappetta used to wear a surgical mask while he was running in lower Manhattan. After he finished his run, the mask looked much like a handkerchief after you've smoked a cigarette through it. Despite this evidence, no other New York runners took up the practice. It seems that running in the street in your underwear is bad enough; wearing a mask is just too much.

Q: I have heard that specific diets and vitamins can protect an individual from the effects of air pollution. What do you think?

A: I am a dietary agnostic. I am unwilling to change my diet on any evidence presented thus far. However, I am a great believer in cod liver oil and its effects on everything, particularly the bronchial tubes. And this may be one area where vitamin E has a protective action. Overall, however, I would say that you are on your own if you think that you have found the answer to air pollution by taking something by mouth.

Q: Is it possible that running leads to a natural protection against air pollution?

A: You can look at it that way. For one thing, once you start to run, you almost always stop smoking, a far more serious problem than air pollution. Also, you develop a much greater pulmonary and cardiac function, so you are able to handle more carbon monoxide. Whether your tolerance to particles and smog will improve, I leave to your individual experiment.

Q: And your final word?

A: I think the benefits of running in the city far outweigh any theoretical disadvantages. The benefits are immediate and evident. The disadvantages seem to be merely threats about the future. In fact, I see no hard evidence that running in an urban setting causes any long-term harm to runners.

For myself, I am all for clean air and clean water, if only for the aesthetics. But I find the present planet no threat, whether rural or urban. A road is a road is a road, whether surrounded by trees or in downtown Chicago or Seattle or Boston.

If by chance I am in a world in which the fittest survive, then I am doing the very best thing I should.

HIGH ALTITUDE

Q: For 27 years, I lived at sea level but am now living at 9200 feet. Could you give me some information on training at different elevations?

A: The main difficulty with training at elevation is in the beginning. Altitude sickness is a frequent occurrence at an elevation of 9200 feet. However, once past this hurdle, the training can be quite similar to that at sea level.

Chapter 37
Surface and Terrain

RUNNING ON GRASS

Q: Shortly after I began running on the streets, I experienced pain in the back of my knee. It eventually spread to my other leg and to the front of both knees and thighs. Then, I started running on grass surfaces and the pain disappeared. But recently, while still on grass, it has returned. What can be done?

A: I found when I played tennis that a set on asphalt would finish my legs but that I could play on grass all day. Grass, however, does tend to be uneven and does cause changes in footstrike that could cause knee problems. In addition, you may have a basic biomechanical problem in your foot that needs some special support. Many runners with pain in the back of the knee have very high arches. Finally, exercises to stretch the Achilles and hamstring muscles may be valuable to you.

ON THE LEVEL

Q: According to the "law of use and disuse," if you don't use a muscle it will atrophy. Some athletes train on mountain trails and other uneven surfaces to insure that all muscles are exercised under varying stresses. Why, then, do you discourage training on uneven surfaces, saying that the uneven footstrike will cause unwanted stresses and possible breakdown elsewhere?

A: I have infrequently run on extremely uneven pasture land and always regretted it. Five miles invariably produced painful knees, and frequently sore arches and ankles as well. Nothing is gained by this. You do not eventually strengthen one set of muscles or make another more flexible. You just stress the foot-leg complex and search out your inherent weaknesses.

Hill work has a lot going for it, but curing inherent structural instability is not one of its benefits. Muscle balancing and flexibility are best attained through regular daily exercises such as the Magic Six (described in Chapter 12).

HARD SURFACES

Q: Six of us run from 6-8 miles during our lunch hour. The course is concrete. On weekends, when we have the opportunity, we run 12-18 miles on paved roads. Four of the six runners are experiencing knee problems—i.e., stiffness and sharp pains in the joints. Our questions are: (1) Does a concrete running surface cause knee problems; (2) what do you suspect the knee problem is; (3) what can be done about it?

A: Given normal feet and arches, the relative hardness of the surface relates directly only to muscle fatigue. The problem of shock has not yet been worked out, but a short gliding style plus sufficient cushioning in shoes can handle almost any surface.

Most runners use roads and handle the shock well. However, if you have an arch or foot problem, long distances on concrete will cause the foot to decompensate (flatten or pronate, which is to say run over on the inside). This transmits a torque of 6-7 degrees to the knee. The result is that the kneecap moves to the side instead of sliding up and down in the groove, and the underside of the kneecap rubs on the knob of the thigh bone. This condition is known as "runner's knee" (technically, "chondromalacia").

The treatment is correct foot support. You can start with store-bought Dr. Scholl's longitudinal arch. But many runners need a full-foot mold.

One other point: The crown of the road can cause difficulty with the foot nearer the center. Running with traffic will throw you over on the inside of the left foot and to the outside of the right one, giving you pain in the left knee. Simply crossing over to run against traffic (or vice versa if your problem is in your right foot) may be sufficient, along with the standard drugstore arches, to give you relief.

DOWNHILL STRAIN

Q: After speaking with a number of runners following the 1976 Boston Marathon, I learned that many were afflicted with tightened quadriceps muscles. In my case, it was the lack of proper training (foot injuries resulted in inadequate mileage during the month and a half prior to the race).

I would appreciate your analysis of why there were so many sore quads. Was it because of the heat and continual hosing down? In past races, my main problems were tightening of the calves, but this time it was the quads.

A: We oldtimers have learned annually of the effect of the Boston Marathon course on the quadriceps. The "checking" of going downhill in the early stages, the long downhill at Lower Newton Falls and then the climb through Newton puts tremendous strain on the quads.

Usually, this becomes apparent as you descend from Boston College, and then you feel it on every slight decline until the finish.

I find that for three days or so after Boston I have to go downstairs backward. Any I doubt that I am alone in this misery.

So it's the course that does it, not heat or humidity. Boston is the supreme test for your quadriceps muscles.

INDOOR PAIN

Q: With the severe winter weather, I sometimes find myself running on an indoor track. After running seven or eight miles on the track, I noticed a pain in the middle of my left calf. I thought it was just a cramp and kept on running. After about three more laps, I knew it was more than a cramp because I couldn't raise myself up on the ball of my foot without excruciating pain. I am certain that the tight curves and pushing off, going around the curves with my left leg is the cause of the problem. I would be interested to know if there are individuals who have similar problems.

A: Indoor running apparently stresses the left (inner) leg, whereas road running stresses the right leg (uppermost on the crest of the road).

However, I have also discovered that activities other than running, even walking for instance, can lead to injuries. Given a weak foot and short, inflexible muscles, the runner has to be very careful that he doesn't exceed his stress limit.

FEET IN THE SAND

Q: I'm employed as an ocean lifeguard. I'm curious whether running on soft sand with or without shoes is a good practice. I generally run about four miles on soft sand without shoes. Would it be a better practice for me to run with shoes on harder sand?

A: Sand gives natural support to the feet. Very hard sand might, however, cause foot strain. You would have to be the judge of that.

I find that it is not the sand but the slant down to the water that gives me trouble. This pronates or flattens the uppermost foot, and causes foot and knee pain.

PART TEN:

PSYCHOLOGICAL FACTORS

"Fitness has to be fun. If it is not play,
there will be no fitness."

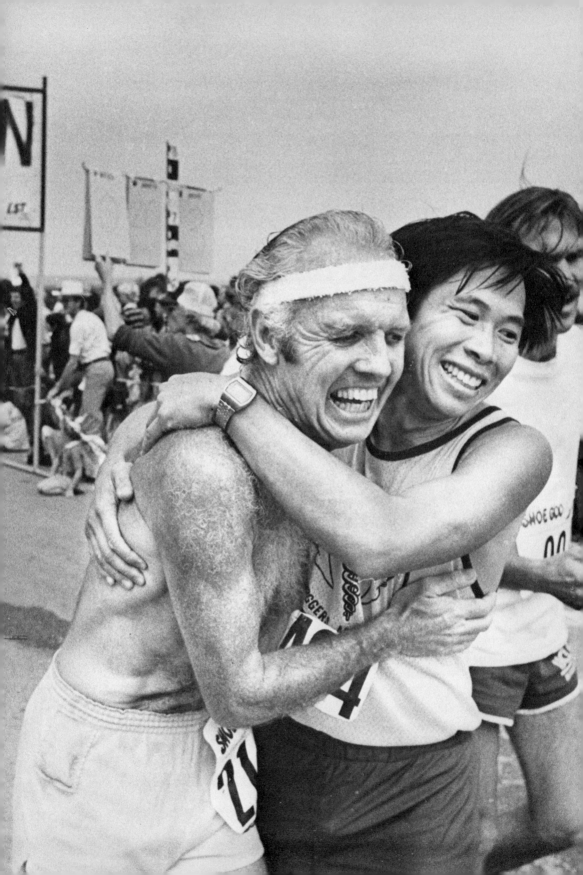

Chapter 38
The Shape You're In

Fitness has to be fun. If it is not play, there will be no fitness. Play, you see, is the process; fitness is merely the product.

What we need, then, is not another "how-to" manual on physical fitness. The mechanics of fitness are absurdly simple. The physiology of fitness could be described on the head of a pin. Yet each month someone in some scientific journal must "prove" that 30-60 minutes of vigorous exercise every other day will convert a spectator into an athlete.

We know this. Everybody knows this. What nobody apparently knows, however, is the *psychology* of fitness, and why people persist at running, swimming, skiing and weight lifting with the intensity usually reserved for converting heathens and staging revolutions.

We need a book to explain not only this intensity but the individuality of its application; why some people must play alone and others are only happy with others; why some people need to hit and be hit while others hate to be touched; why winning and losing are important to some and of no consequence to others. We need a book to give us physical education guidance much like the vocational guidance we received in arriving at our careers.

Fortunately, such a book—actually a series of books—exists. They outline the theory and practice of constitutional psychology developed by Dr. William Sheldon. This psychology supposes that our function follows our structure. It continues in "the persistent tradition that the shape of a man promises certain traits in his temperament"—that fat men are jolly and thin men dour and muscular men not averse to mixing it up with their fists.

Sheldon accepted this idea of the determination of the temperament and the personality from the body build, but then went further. He discovered the three basic body components and devised a method to measure their contribution to the total structure. This he called the "somatotype." He then took these various body types and correlated them with the three basic components of temperament.

These three were already a part of our inherited wisdom. We already knew you could look at a person and tell whether he was made for fight, flight or negotiation. We could tell which one of our friends was an extrovert and which was an introvert. We could divide those we met into doers, thinkers and talkers.

All this is simply common sense which we apply every day. Sheldon turned that common sense into a science. He took measurements that established which of the three layers of the human embryo was dominant in the individual being examined.

Those three layers are the "endoderm," the source of the intestine and abdominal contents; the "mesoderm," the source of the bones and muscles; and the "ectoderm," which forms the hair, skin, nails and nervous system. Whichever tissue dominates gives a person a characteristic body build and a temperament to go with it.

• *Endomorphs* have large intestinal tracts and tend to be spherical in shape. They have heavy bodies which are wider through the abdomen than across the chest. They like to eat and drink and socialize, and when under stress they seek other people. Their main assets are good insulation and the ability to float. They are best suited to sports that do not call for speed and strength—swimming, cycling, skiing, walking, jogging, tennis, golf or bowling, for instance. Endomorphs need company. They are Pickwickian extroverts.

• *Mesomorphs* are also extroverts. They, however, are strong, muscular people who are natural athletes. Their extroversion is the desire to compete, to go head-to-head with an opponent. They like contact sports and like to hit something or somebody. Mesomorphs tend to be courageous, adventurous, noisy and have a Spartan indifference to pain. They are happy with the martial arts, wrestling, boxing and the hitting games. They prefer energetic games involving skill and danger. They can be induced into running, cycling or the like if they can add the challenge of personal goals.

• *Ectomorphs* tend to be skinny, fragile, linear people with a low threshold for pain, both physical and psychic. They are anti-social, dislike noise and confusion and body contact. They are natural loners and are most happy by themselves. Should they compete, they prefer contests where the other players are simply witnesses to what they do. They know that the world needs endomorphs but would rather not have them in the immediate vicinity. The ectomorph, therefore, is the ideal lonely long-distance runner, cross-country skier or walker.

BODY TYPES

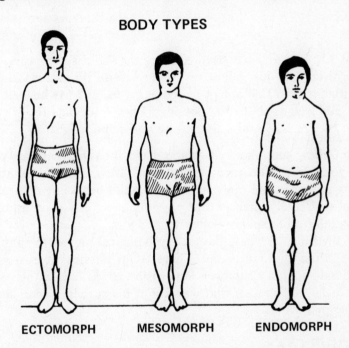

ECTOMORPH   MESOMORPH   ENDOMORPH

Now, we know that we are made for our sport, made for our play. We have the body to do some things better than others, and a temperament that tells us how and with whom. We must listen to the message from our cells, the tune our body-mind is singing. Only then will we be authentic and find our true play. Only then will we discover the "why" behind every successful fitness program.

Chapter 39
Running and the Head

SIZE

Q: My husband has been running for about seven years. No long distances—just about two miles several times a week. My question is this: Can a man be too heavy to run? My husband is 6'1" and weighs about 190 pounds. When I see pictures of runners, they're all so thin. Should he lose some weight?

A: A few years back, I would have thought your husband was too big a man to enjoy running. Now, I'm not so sure. There are more and more men of his build becoming dedicated runners. Usually, men of that physique are fairly good athletes and prefer other sports—often team sports.

If anything, he would have a psychological barrier to running rather than a physical one. There is no physical reason your husband shouldn't run even long distances, as long as his exercise is play. If he feels that way about his running, you should be happy.

WITHDRAWAL

Q: I keep hearing that people who run regularly for years will have to "taper off" slowly if they ever decide to quit. Is there any truth in this?

A: All that happens to a runner who stops is that in 4-6 weeks he becomes deconditioned. At that point, he is little different in most respects from his neighbor of the same age and build. He has simply lost certain endurance ability. He does not suffer from any other problems, except perhaps in sleep loss and nervousness due to withdrawal.

DEPRESSION

Q: I am a runner who has been laid up for six months. The physical problem is being cared for, but I've found it hard to adjust mentally.

Running is my life. I used it as an outlet for everything, as well as for meeting and getting to know new people. More important, it provided me with the time and ability to think.

My head got stale as I sat through the longest summer of my life. I soon found myself in a deep state of depression. I tried swimming but found it no comfort. I can now run a short distance, which at times helps and at times teases. What can a runner do to avoid this kind of mental rut when stuck spectating?

A: Read Ecclesiastes, I suppose. I find swimming to be a real clock-watching bore.

Cycling seems to be the best alternative. Race walking is practically injury free and seems to have people much like us. Cross-country skiing is something I never tried, but seems to interest others.

But, as you say, nothing does it like running, and I have no real answer to your question.

EXTREMES

Q: My husband runs to work, eight miles one way. After about the third day of this running pattern, he becomes hell on wheels. He becomes violent, obnoxious, cruel, disrespectful. You name it, he does it. Can you shed some light on this problem?

A: Running is a stressful activity, and can be carried to extremes. One reaction to this may be an accentuation of any psychological tendency to depression, and presumably to agitation, paranoia or schizophrenia.

It seems to me your husband's reactions have become abnormal. What he needs is a complete rest from running to see if this is the cause of his problems. I doubt, however, that he will stop unless he gets injured or somehow hears that a 2-4-week layoff sometimes does wonders.

NEUROSES

Q: As a runner being treated with psychotherapy for long-simmering neuroses in addition to more recently acquired marital problems, I'm wondering about the possible causal relationships among these factors: exercise, diet, metabolism and mental health. When I finally decided to seek treatment, it coincided with a very fatiguing race—the only one I had ever entered. Could the running have suddenly altered my metabolism enough that neuroses resulted or were aggravated?

A: The subjects you touch on have been inadequately researched, and this is not for lack of trying. Almost daily, we see articles on the effects of exercise and diet on the emotions and metabolism, the significance of low blood sugar and the role of exhaustion.

Unfortunately, those results will not stand scientific analysis, and we are left as experiments of one to try megavitamins, macrobiotic diets, etc.

For myself, I lean toward depletion and exhaustion as our major stresses. Many of us can train only two to three times a week on a consistent basis to stay well. Many of us need naps every day, and are actually made for a four-hour work day and a four-day work week. Over-extended, we go to the edges of our personality and beyond.

I can see this in myself. Sleep, naps, running only Tuesdays, Thursdays and Sundays, and occasionally some vitamin B-12 make things look brighter.

THE JITTERS

Q: I am 33 years old and have been running long distance for two years. I lost 90 pounds. I drink coffee and eat high-cholesterol foods. I train 10-14 miles daily. I am a nervous person and take five milligrams of Valium, especially when I drink coffee. I tried to break off the Valium for a week and drank no coffee, and I got a tight feeling in my chest and very nervous. Are these withdrawal symptoms from taking nerve medicine? How can drinking coffee and then popping Valium to relax me be harmful to my heart or nervous system?

A: Usually, the long-distance training will get you off Valium. However, coffee is another story. I have tried to quit drinking it but always come back. At times, I use tea and can avoid those coffee jitters, but usually I just give in and go with coffee.

Gandhi said never to give up anything until it was no longer necessary. You'll know when you don't need either of these.

RELAXATION

Herbert Benson of Harvard suggests a "non-cultic" form of relaxation similar to transcendental meditation in its effects but without TM's mystical trappings.

1. Sit quietly in a comfortable position.

2. Close your eyes.

3. Deeply relax all your muscles, beginning with your feet and progressing up to your face. Keep them deeply relaxed.

4. Breathe through your nose. Become aware of your breathing. As you breathe out, say the word "one" silently. For example, breathe in...out, "one"; in...out, "one"; etc.

5. Continue for 20 minutes. You may open your eyes to check the time, but do not use an alarm. When you finish, sit quietly for several minutes—at first with closed eyes and later with open eyes.

6. Do not worry about whether you are successful in achieving a deep level of relaxation. Maintain a passive attitude and permit relaxation to occur at its own pace. When distracting thoughts occur, ignore them and continue repeating "one." With practice, the response should come with little effort.

Practice the technique twice daily, but not within two hours after a meal since the digestive processes seem to interfere with the elicitation of anticipated changes.

"PSYCHING"

Q: I'm a high school cross-country runner. This past season, I've had mental trouble getting myself ready for meets. I am physically prepared to run better races, but am not mentally prepared. Could you tell me a good method of preparing for a big race without over-psyching?

A: The primary rule in racing is to run intelligently—i.e., to run a race with a general plan as to pace and how you are going to adjust to the other runners' tactics. It's my guess that most poor races are because of poor planning rather than poor psyching.

To avoid over-psyching, many athletes use relaxation techniques. Most of these involve attention to slow, deep breathing and relaxation of individual muscle groups.

Under-psyching usually occurs when you are diverted completely from thinking of the race. I try to start thinking about the race about 15 minutes before and shut off conversation. This is difficult when you are seeing old friends and in the holiday atmosphere of the race.

You should develop an attitude that you want to do your best and let winning take care of itself. Our game is the race, not winning. It is a contest in which our fellow runners are not so much opponents as witnesses of what we do.

I psych myself up in order to be the complete runner—to make running, at least for that period, the most important thing in my life. I want to do well, even to win, but I'm not upset when I don't. I find the stopwatch to be my major opponent.

Finally, I would never start thinking about a race the day before. That surely must be self-defeating. When a race seems too important, remember what a football coach told his quarterback before the Rose Bowl: "There are 600 million Chinese who don't even know this game is being played."

Chapter 40
Jogger, Runner, Racer

DIFFERENCES

To the inexperienced eye, the jogger and the runner look much the same. Even to those quite close to these peculiar forms of behavior, the distinction between the two states may be difficult to make. There is, however, a world of difference between the jogger just coming into this activity and the runner who comes out the other end.

These days when everyone's consciousness is being raised, it has become important what you call people. Each age, sex and ethnic group has a favored designation. There are other terms they regard as pejorative and insulting. What you consider appropriate, they might consider an epithet. So there can be some hesitancy when faced with someone in running shoes (if you are still calling them "sneakers," you are in real trouble) in choosing his correct label.

My initial reflex after 15 years at this game was to define a runner as "a jogger who has entered a race." The essential difference between a jogger and a runner, to me, was not ability or training. I know joggers who train longer and can run faster than runners who compete. It was the attitude, the perception of self, the need for a different expression that led the jogger to fill out that first entry blank and take the giant step into competition.

Now, I'm not so sure about that definition. The jogger who goes into races becomes a racer, not a runner. The jogger has merely become a competitor, a change that may be more sidewise than forward in progressing toward the goal of becoming a runner.

THE JOGGER

The jogger and the racer are in many ways quite alike. If the jogger is a runner in embryo, so is the racer. If the jogger is a novice, it is also true of the racer.

For each, the growth is first in ability. For the jogger, the yards become miles, the minutes become hours, the days become weeks. The dedicated pursuit of fitness occupies his mind and will. Jogging is the perfecting of the body. It ends there.

Some see the jogger as an automaton. "Jogging is a form of exercise," write Drs. Roseman and Friedman in their treatise on Type-A personalities, "in which man transforms himself into a machine, chug-chug-chugging along looking neither right nor left."

William Zinsser of the *New York Times* described joggers as "self-contained prisoners of fitness." He could see, he said, no joy on their faces, only duty and pain.

It is true, of course, that the jogger is looking for results. Joggers expect to firm the body, lose weight, develop their legs, improve their wind. They want to get back into shape. It is also true that it is not easy, particularly at first. The muscles protest. Fatigue becomes manifest. Running is a chore and frequently a depressing one, in much the same way the student of Zen finds the lotus position at first impossible. Eventually, of course, it becomes quite natural—in fact, the preferred attitude.

Eventually, the jogger finds his nice slow pace, that comfortable level, settles into it and relaxes. At that point, the jogger becomes content. There is no need to go farther. Good things are happening to his body. There is a perceptible difference in energy, in the waistline, in the response to tension and aggravation.

The jogger has found the way to accomplish the most in the least amount of time, then fills that quota day after day. Here at last is the way to dissipate stress, the method of handling a zero-sum society where someone always wins and, therefore, others always have to lose. The jogger has discovered that the fittest do survive and has found a way to that fitness.

But if the jogger is goal-oriented, so is the racer. The jogger has in mind correcting the physical effects of the sedentary life. The racer, on the other hand, is interested in remedying the psychological effects of that life: the boredom, the lack of self-esteem, the apathy, the depression, the loss of interest. Only later will they both see that the runner, without directly willing or seeking it, fills in the defects of our spiritual life.

Most people begin as joggers, then become racers and finally grow to the status of runner. It seems to me that this is the normal progression, although others go from being joggers to runners without ever entering a race.

THE RACER

I had been a racer in college and always thought of myself as a runner. Yet I recall in those four years at school only once running just for the fun of it—one day running in the hills for enjoyment.

So when I began again 15 years ago, I had no more hint about the truth of running than the other novice, the jogger. I began as a racer and only much later became a runner. Only much later did I come to see running in perspective. I began much like the jogger.

"To jog," says Webster, "is to run at a slow, leisurely, monotonous pace." I did just that on the 10-lap-to-the-mile track I laid out in my backyard. It was some time before I was willing to let anyone see me running the roads in my shorts and T-shirt. A runner in those days was a rare sight and an object of curiosity, if not ridicule.

In time, I increased my mileage and pace, and took to the roads. I was still a jogger by the standards of the National Jogging Association because my pace was slower than seven minutes per mile. But I was by then a racer. I had found a new world.

I had started the project because I needed a goal as a substitute for others that had failed. Joggers run for a different purpose. They may find jogging mindless, boring and time-consuming. But they are willing to do it for the sake of fitness. Jogging complements a full life, but they have other paths to fulfillment.

For me, it was a life that was mindless and boring and time-consuming. I was racing to make it different. What I needed was something to satisfy ego, something that would set me apart, something that would justify me—even if it were as absurb as a person my age training for a mile race.

I pursued the five-minute mile with the persistence of Ahab chasing the white whale. I ran race after race after race. Then, I got into longer and longer races. In time, I added the sub-three-hour marathon to my goals. All the while, I was learning more and more about myself, and discovering again and again the satisfactions, the joys, the sense of a job well done that comes from the race.

Once experienced, the race becomes all. When I began racing, the family lost me. Every Sunday, I was on the highway looking for competition. One Sunday, I ran a 5000-meter race in New York City and then traveled down to Philadelphia for a nine-mile race that evening. There were times in the summer when I ran as many as three races a week.

Racing was in many ways a revelation. I found I was capable of things I wouldn't have dreamed of attempting before, and that I was full of misconceptions about myself and others. The race was a place where I learned how to handle pain and give an improbable effort, and do it all alone. Yet at the end I discovered that each of us racers had done the same. We were all brothers and sisters, and each of us commoners was a hero.

Why race? For all of the above reasons, I suppose, plus others: the need to be tested, perhaps; the need to take risks; the chance to be number one.

THE RUNNER

I am not sure when I became a runner. One thing is certain: It came long after I began racing. For years, racing possessed me. I would go anywhere for a race and even farther for a medal or a trophy. That feeling is still not extinguished. But now I am a racer who has become a runner.

Racing is the lovemaking of the runner. It is an excitement in the blood. There is the same agitation, the same stirring of the pulse, the same feeling in the chest, the same delightful apprehension you feel when nearing the one you love.

But there is also an element of fear. If racing attracts, it also repels. As I try for my perfection, I am all too aware of my imperfections. When I race, I am the person William James called twice-born. Such people see an element of real wrong in the world, especially in themselves. And they know this must be overcome by doing something heroic, that they themselves must be cleansed by suffering.

I accept that. I still seek the race, seek to be tested, ask to meet pain and pass or fail. The difference now is that the race has simply become a race. I continue to race, and I never give less than my best. At the finish, I am on my hands and knees, gasping and thinking this is absurd. But I have put aside the winning and the losing, the getting of trophies and not getting trophies. I have had my fill of that. I have become a runner.

Jogging, they say, is competing against yourself. Racing is competing against others. Running is discovering that competition is only competing. It is essential and not essential. It is important and not important. Running is finally seeing everything in perspective. Running is discovering the wholeness, the unity that everyone seeks. Running is the fusion of body, mind and soul in that beautiful relaxation that joggers and racers find so difficult to achieve.

Relaxation is the sign of the runner, not the racer or jogger. Somewhere along the way, I learned to relax. I learned to relax not only my body, but my mind and soul as well. I discovered that running is an art form and that I could be the running as the dancer is the dance. I found that running is play—and even more, a sort of spiritual discipline. It is a way of seeing reality, of perceiving the good and the true. Running gives me my special perspective.

"Each of us has a mission of truth," wrote Ortega. "What my eye sees of reality is seen by no other eye. We are irreplaceable; we are necessary."

When I run, truly run, I am certain of that. It is all there. My body does what it does best. The mind like a kaleidoscope constantly rearranges the things it has stored into new and exciting patterns. And my soul utterly loses itself in the present.

The runner has a view of life that makes all the jogging and racing worthwhile.

Chapter 41
Living with Pain

LISTEN TO YOURSELF

One of the basic rules of health is "Listen to your body." I am responsible for my health, and to respond to my body I must listen to it, learn from it. I must, as Thoreau wrote, occupy my body with delight, its weariness and its refreshments.

Listening to my body means listening to every aspect: learning what delights it, what disagrees with it; learning what to eat, what not to eat; learning how much sleep I need and when it is helpful to nap; learning how best to breathe and what is the most economical running form.

There are, to be sure, negative signals as well as positive ones. Some of the symptoms of danger are subtle. They are deeply hidden and go unheeded. Others, like vomiting and diarrhea, urinating blood and an attack of asthma, palpitation of the heart and giant hives, get our attention immediately. One of the more ominous of these warnings is pain. Pain anywhere, however mild, is a cause of concern, and its continuance is a source of anxiety and even alarm.

Fortunately, pain has certain characteristics which help us establish its cause and implications: where it is, when it occurs, what makes it worse, what makes it better, the presence or absence of tenderness, whether it occurs running or not running, whether it is worse going up hill or downhill, jogging or sprinting, in certain shoes and not in others. All help in the diagnosis and treatment.

This is especially true of injuries of the lower extremities in runners. When I have pain in the foot, leg, knee, thigh, groin or low back, I listen to my body and try to answer two questions:

The first is, *"Should I run with it?"* The general rule is "run through annoyance but not pain." I have a pain threshold at the level of a firm handshake, so I adhere strictly to this rule. Annoyance is safe. Pain means "Stop!" I let my body tell me.

I have had knee pains and muscle pulls that have stopped me in my tracks. So I have limped to the nearest phone and waited for a lift for home.

On the other hand, I have used running to answer the second question, *"What is causing this pain?"* Running with annoyance and through it is one of the better ways to come up with a diagnosis. I use the road as a laboratory. I can establish the type of shoe that helps. I can run pigeontoed and see if this helps. I can change the side of the road and do much the same. I can run with my toes floating and take my shin muscles out of the action. I can get up on my toes and determine how much heel strike is entering into the picture.

There is much to be learned in action. I can also evaluate the effect of a drugstore arch support in my shoe, or using a heel lift first on the good side then on the bad. I know of one runner who reversed his store-bought arch supports, put the right one in the left shoe and the left in the right and obtained relief. This is do-it-yourself medicine no physician would have thought of.

The road has become my examining room. I take my aching body for a run so I can learn what is going on and how to cure it. If I have a pain in my buttocks and wonder whether it is my sciatica or my chronically recurring hamstring injury, I can find out on the nearest hill. Going uphill bothers the hamstring, whereas that bentover position favors the sciatica. Going downhill does the reverse. The swayback position puts the sciatic nerve on the stretch and eases the pull on the hamstring muscle. Speed work, I have discovered, is bad for both. The stride-out gets the hamstring, the pushoff bends the spine backward on the sciatic roots.

If I get pain on the outside of my leg, I begin to wonder if my arch supports are overcorrected. Pain on the outside of the leg, knee and hip seems to be due to shock and too much control of the foot. So I remove the arch and run without it to see what happens. What happens usually is the pain on the side of my leg leaves, only to be replaced by pain in the Achilles tendon. I have lost the extra four millimeters of heel that arch support gives me, and I evidently need it.

Sometimes, that four millimeters is not enough. The Achilles pain gets chronic. Then, I keep inserting felt under the heel until I can run in comfort. Sometimes, the felt pad is so high, my foot is almost out of the shoe. Never mind; the truth is what works, not what they say in the books. When I work with my body, I am an architect, a carpenter, a mason. I am also learning things that are not yet in the texts—ideas and concepts that are still part of an oral tradition.

I have been running for more than 15 years, and for most of those years I have been trying to tell other physicians what I have discovered on the roads. Now, I limit my advice to those who are out running on their roads themselves and are listening to their bodies.

ILLOGICAL, IRRATIONAL, IMPORTANT

A physician wrote to the *New York Times* complaining about my annual column on the Boston Marathon. He'd had enough, said he, of Dr. Sheehan's clap-trap glorifying pain. It was clear to him that pain is something we must avoid. Anyone who revels in it, as I apparently do, is obviously in need of psychotherapy.

He is right. There is no sense to pain. It is nonsense to glorify it, absurd to look for it in a marathon, and then feel purified and cleansed as a result. The perfect life, it would appear, is pain-free. To seek pain is illogical; to endure it, irrational; to extent it, insane.

The doctor's position is logical, rational and totally sane. Why get involved with pain?

But I am a runner. I have lived with pain. I see things differently. When the doctor feels pain, he knows he's doing something wrong. When I feel pain, I know I'm doing something right. Pain teaches, shapes, strengthens and develops the person I am. The runner in me accepts this. I know that pain is the only means I have for doing and knowing my best.

For me, the evil of suffering is cured by more suffering. I must not avoid it. I must embrace it. I have to back pain into a corner and possess it, control it. With it, I make payment for the person I was and make an offering to the person I will be.

"What then is man?" asks Victor Frankl, a psychiatrist who survived Dachau and Auschwitz. He then answers, "We have learned to know him in the camps...where what remained was man himself melted down in the white heat of suffering and pain to the essentials, to the human himself."

I am, you will say, presumptuous to compare what happens in a marathon to those terrible ordeals, yet the truth is there. Courage and bravery and pain are inseparable wherever they occur. Whatever the circumstance, it is the work done, love loved and suffering suffered that we end up being proud of. And nowhere in the runner's life are work and love and suffering more apparent than in that "acme of athletic heroism," the marathon.

At Boston in 1978, I entered the final miles with the pain gradually rising like a tide over my body—and along with it a feeling of apprehension about my daughter Sarah somewhere behind me, running her first marathon. Then, on the final hill I came up behind this paraplegic man in a wheelchair.

It was, of course, insane for that brave young man to be pushing himself in a wheelchair that marathon distance. Yet there he was, struggling desperately up that crowd-lined hill, paying for every inch with painful agonized thrusts of his arms and shoulders.

Then, the crowd took up a chant, "Do it! Do it!" each time he grasped the wheels and pushed forward. And so it became a hill we all climbed, those hundreds shouting and caring, and the young man and all the runners around him. The world became those few yards on a Newton hill where we all shared in that pain, and then the joy when he crested the hill and before him lay the downhill and Boston and glory.

Later, after I finished and had first fallen asleep in the tub and taken my turn in the bed, the room began to fill with happy, worn-out runners. Then, the real waiting began. It did not end until the bell rang, they opened the door, and there stood Sarah, pale and spent and shaken and utterly beautiful. She stood there, no more than what she wore and what she had become, one of the 5000 heroes in the Boston Marathon.

The doctor is right. Pain is irrational, illogical and unexplainable. So he sees no reason to live with it.

Those of us who ran at Boston have the opposite problem. We can't live without it.

Ailment Index

Running ailments come from multiple causes and show multiple symptoms. So it is impossible to separate them neatly into chapters. This index helps combine the information spread through the book. It lists problem areas by *chapter*. For more details, see the full index at the back of the book.

Medical Advice Index

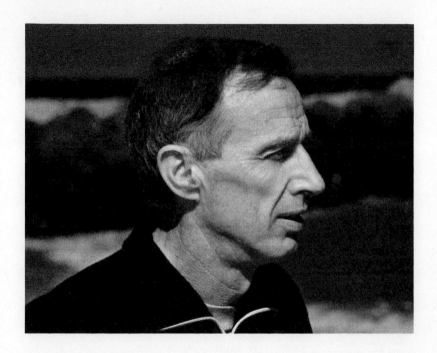

About the Author

George Sheehan, M.D., combines a unique spread of talents: doctor, runner, thinker, writer.

A cardiologist practicing in Red Bank, N.J., Sheehan returned to running at age 45. He once held the world mile record for runners 50 and older, and he still competes regularly at distances up to the marathon.

Sheehan writes on both medical and philosophical topics for a number of publications, notably *Runner's World* for which he serves as medical editor.

His earlier books are *Dr. Sheehan on Running* (World Publications, 1975) and *Running and Being: The Total Experience* (Simon and Schuster, 1978). The latter was a national bestseller.

Sheehan and his wife Mary Jane, parents of 12 children, live in Rumson, N.J.